D1026314

ASTAXANTHIN

Natural Astaxanthin: King of the Carotenoids

By Bob Capelli
with Dr. Gerald Cysewski

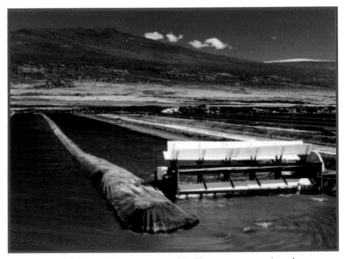

Natural Astaxanthin concentrated in Haematococcus microalgae

Published by Cyanotech Corporation
© Copyright 2007 by Cyanotech Corporation
Second printing 2008
All rights reserved.

ISBN-13: 978-0-9792353-0-6
ISBN-10: 0-9792353-0-8

Publisher's Note

The information here is for educational purposes only; it is not to be taken as medical advice or as an attempt to sell a particular product. The opinions expressed are those of the authors. People with medical problems or questions should consult a health professional. Information in this book is not intended to diagnose, treat, cure or prevent any disease.

The publisher of this book, Cyanotech Corporation, is a producer of Natural Astaxanthin from Haematococcus microalgae. Cyanotech sponsored several of the studies in this book, but wishes to make it clear that none of the animal studies were sponsored by Cyanotech. Our company policy is to sponsor medical research as human clinical trials, exclusively with subjects recruited as willing volunteers. We do not condone animal experimentation; yet animal studies done by others are reported in this book in order that the reader may fully understand the ongoing medical research and the potential benefits of Astaxanthin in human nutrition.

This book may not be reproduced in whole or in part, by any means, without written permission from Cyanotech Corporation, 73-4460 Queen Kaahumanu Highway, Suite 102, Kailua-Kona, HI 96740 USA.

This book is dedicated to the scientists who study, the nutritionists who recommend and the consumers who believe in Natural Astaxanthin, as well as to those willing to take the time to read this book to learn about this wonderful nutrient. Also, to all the people who work at Cyanotech Corporation, the worldwide leader in Natural Astaxanthin research and production, particularly the hard working, loyal people who work on our Production Team in the hot Hawaiian sun to produce the algae from which Natural Astaxanthin is extracted—your work is greatly appreciated! Special thanks must also be given to Nicholle Davis for her help in proofreading and formatting the references, to Susie Cysewski for her outstanding graphic artistry and to Barbara Lewis for her final proofreading with her eagle eye. Lastly, to my wife for putting up with me for almost 20 years.

Bob Capelli
Holualoa, Hawaii
November 2006

Table of Contents

Introduction

We are just beginning to understand the wonderful health benefits that Natural Astaxanthin (pronounced asta-ZAN-thin) can bring to humans, as well as animals. While many studies have already been done, there is still potential for a great deal more to be discovered. I foresee a time not too long from now when Astaxanthin (although difficult to pronounce) becomes a household word. For twenty years I have been involved with natural supplements and herbs, and I have to say that I have never been as excited about any other natural product as I am about Natural Astaxanthin. Scientists have not found any substance that has stronger antioxidant effects for free radical elimination or singlet oxygen quenching. And as the impressive anti-inflammatory properties of Astaxanthin become more widely researched and recognized, a whole new channel for the use of Astaxanthin in human nutrition is opening. Medical researchers are finding links between inflammation and a myriad of life threatening and debilitating diseases. The necessity of combating this "silent inflammation" is becoming more apparent each year. At the same time, scientists continue to prove that supplementing with antioxidants is essential to lengthening and improving the quality of our lives.

As people begin to supplement with Astaxanthin, they report physical differences—less pains from arthritis, a better workout with quicker recovery, extra energy, less colds and flu, and the ability to stay in the sun longer without getting sunburned. They tell their families and friends and then, their families and friends try it and they too feel results. We've seen in Hawaii where we first introduced BioAstin® Natural Astaxanthin eight years ago how this can snowball. Generally, in the mainland states, Natural Astaxanthin can only be found in health food stores. But in Hawaii, you can walk into Wal-Mart or Costco where they have 10 – 20 cases stacked at all times, or stop in most local supermarkets or drug stores to purchase a bottle. The per capita use of Natural Astaxanthin in Hawaii is extremely high and still growing, and this has happened without much advertising—simply through word of mouth and doctor recommendations.

Someday, I believe that all good multivitamins will contain Natural Astaxanthin, and that softgel capsules with Natural Astaxanthin will be taken by as many people as now consume Vitamin C. In the meantime I urge everyone to read this short book, weigh the evidence to date, and decide for yourself if you should try a bottle.

Bob Capelli
September 2006

CHAPTER 1

"King of the Carotenoids"

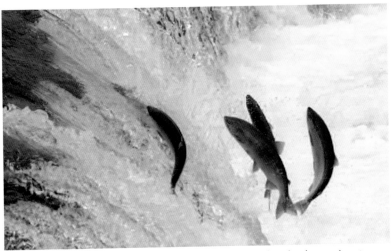

Salmon's upstream marathon: The greatest display of strength and endurance in nature

Have you ever seen a salmon swimming upstream? Look at the size of the salmon above and compare their size to the force of the water coming down the river at them.

Now think about this—Salmon continue swimming up these raging rivers for up to seven days.

Let's put this into human perspective: Take a six foot tall man and have him swim against 30 foot waves for a week straight and be able to reach his destination which is 100 miles away.

How is it possible that salmon can make this heroic swim, which certainly is the greatest athletic feat in nature? Natural Astaxanthin.

Natural Astaxanthin is found in the highest concentration in the animal kingdom in the muscles of salmon, and scientists theorize that this is what allows them to complete this epic swim. We have long known that exercise causes a

1

great amount of oxidation in the muscles. So by concentrating the strongest antioxidant, Natural Astaxanthin in the muscles, the oxidation is thus prevented and the salmon are capable of doing something that seems almost impossible.

We certainly don't want anyone to think that because we make the analogy with humans above that we're suggesting that you run out to the health food store, buy a bottle of Natural Astaxanthin and then try to swim from New York to Paris. But there is certainly sufficient evidence, both from testimonials and scientific studies, that taking 4 – 8 mg of Natural Astaxanthin per day will provide greater strength and endurance.

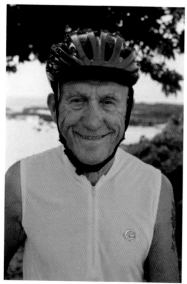

Max Burdick, 78 year old triathlete and avid Natural Astaxanthin user

One story we love to tell at Cyanotech, the world's largest producer of Natural Astaxanthin, is of Max Burdick. Max is an Ironman triathlete. For those of you who aren't familiar with triathlons, this is an endurance sporting event where participants swim for 2.4 miles (3.9 km) and then bicycle for 112 miles (180 km). Then, instead of falling down exhausted in a hammock and taking a nap like most normal humans would do, they go out and run a 26.2 mile (42.2 km) marathon.

There are plenty of triathletes—so what's so special about Max Burdick? Max is 78 years old.

Max was competing for years in triathlons but could never seem to finish. Halfway through the bicycling stage his legs would start to burn and he would have to stop. Max discovered BioAstin®, a brand of Natural Astaxanthin, and began supplementing with 2 capsules each day. It was then, at the age of 75, that Max was able to finish a triathlon. He has continued to use BioAstin and finish triathlons for the last three years, and has remained a dedicated Natural Astaxanthin user.

But Natural Astaxanthin isn't just for helping older athletes like Max. All types of people may receive benefits like increased energy, greater stamina and improved strength by supplementing with Astaxanthin. People that have busy schedules and would like a natural way to get more out of their day should try it;

weekend warriors who want to recover faster and get back to their real jobs should also try it; and young athletes who want to excel in their sports may also benefit greatly from it.

Another triathlete who swears by Natural Astaxanthin is Tim Marr. Tim

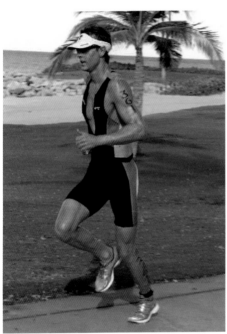

started taking Astaxanthin when he was in college and just beginning to get heavily involved in endurance events. He said that, even with a student's meager finances, he still knew that Natural Astaxanthin was well worth the investment. As of the writing of this book, Tim is 27 years old and just coming into his peak years as a triathlete—and he's winning competitions. Among many other first place finishes, Tim recently won the 2006 Pan American Long Distance Triathlon World Championship. Tim says, "BioAstin is one of my favorite tools as a professional athlete. I want to thank BioAstin for helping me achieve my goals—it's an important part of all my results."

Professional triathlete Tim Marr, among the world's elite in his sport, credits Natural Astaxanthin for helping him to achieve his goals.

But we don't want to focus exclusively on Natural Astaxanthin's benefits for athletes and energy. As we'll learn in the following pages, Natural Astaxanthin does so many things for so many people—the strength and endurance example is only one of the reasons why Natural Astaxanthin is called the "King of the Carotenoids." The many other benefits will become clear as we examine all of the scientific research and read the testimonials of many ecstatic users of Natural Astaxanthin. But first let's talk a little about carotenoids in general.

Other Carotenoids

For those of you who don't know what carotenoids are, chances are you've eaten a few in the last 24 hours. Carotenoids are the pigments that give many of the foods we eat their beautiful colors. That ripe, red tomato you had in your salad last night is red because of a carotenoid called "lycopene." The corn on the cob you had at the company picnic last summer is yellow because of another carotenoid called "zeaxanthin." And of course, the carrots you eat (because you heard as a kid that you should eat carrots to help your eyes because "you've never seen a rabbit with glasses") are orange because of "beta carotene." In fact, "carrots" actually get their name from this famous pigment that makes them orange, "carotene."

Carotenoids are divided into two distinct groups: Members of the first group are called "Carotenes." This is probably the more widely known group because of its most famous member, beta carotene. Some of the other well known carotenes are lycopene and alpha carotene.

The other group, of which Astaxanthin is a proud member, is called "Xanthophylls" (pronounced ZAN-tho-fils). Some other notable xanthophylls are lutein and zeaxanthin. The difference between these two groups is that

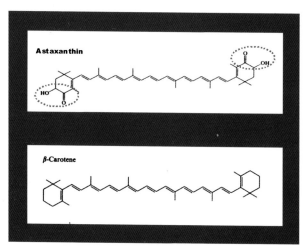

Hydroxyl groups at the end of the Astaxanthin molecule make it very different from beta carotene and other carotenoids

Xanthophylls have hydroxyl groups at the end of the molecules. Astaxanthin has more hydroxyl groups than the other Xanthophylls, which allows it to do more in the human body than its closely-related family members like lutein and zeaxanthin.

On page 4 is a comparison of the Astaxanthin and the beta carotene molecules. You can see that they look similar, except for the ends of the molecule that have the hydroxyl "O" and "OH" groups. This small difference adds up to a huge disparity in terms of functional abilities of these carotenoid cousins.

Some of the many things that Natural Astaxanthin can do that beta carotene (and many other carotenoids) cannot:

1. Cross the blood-brain barrier and bring antioxidant and anti-inflammatory protection to the brain and central nervous system
2. Cross the blood-retinal barrier and bring antioxidant and anti-inflammatory protection to the eyes
3. Travel throughout the body effectively to bring antioxidant and anti-inflammatory protection at a high activity level to all the organs and the skin
4. Span the cell membranes
5. Bond with muscle tissue
6. Work as a super-powerful antioxidant and quickly eliminate free radicals and neutralize singlet oxygen

There are over 700 different carotenoids, although most people have only heard of a few at best. They are produced in nature by plankton, algae and plants as well as a small number of bacteria and fungi. In plants and algae, carotenoids are actually part of the process of photosynthesis along with chlorophyll. Some animals can actually eat a certain carotenoid and then convert it in their body into a different carotenoid, but all animals must originally obtain carotenoids from their diet.

5

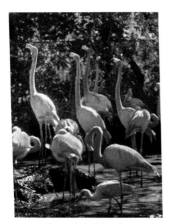
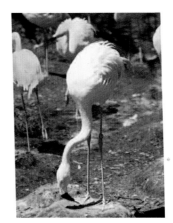

Normal pink flamingos   *A "pink" flamingo that didn't eat its carotenoids*

One example of an animal that can convert carotenoids that it ingests is the pink flamingo. Flamingos eat algae that contain the yellow carotenoid zeaxanthin and the orange carotenoid beta carotene, and then their bodies convert them into the pinkish-red carotenoids Astaxanthin and canthaxanthin. Without carotenoids in their diet, the pink flamingo would be an ugly beige color; and without the ability to convert the carotenoids it eats into Astaxanthin and canthaxanthin, the pink flamingo would be yellowish orange!

Carotenoids have a wonderful ability to interact with and neutralize "oxidants," chemically reactive oxygen species known as singlet oxygen and free radicals. Natural Astaxanthin has the greatest ability to serve in this "anti"-oxidant function, which is why it is the world's strongest natural antioxidant. But many other carotenoids also have an antioxidant effect.

An excellent example of how animals use carotenoids is seen in cold water fish such as salmon and trout. These fish accumulate Astaxanthin from their diets and deposit it in their flesh to protect their tissues and cells from oxidation. This results in the healthy pinkish-red glow you see in fillets of wild salmon or trout. (Many fish farmers use synthetic Astaxanthin to mimic this color in their farmed salmon and trout—more about this unnatural process later.)

Some carotenoids are absolutely necessary for the existence of different species. For example, humans need vitamin A. Vitamin A comes from beta carotene in our diet that the body converts into vitamin A on an as-needed basis. Contrary to high doses of pure Vitamin A which can be toxic, there is no toxicity level for beta carotene.

Beta carotene is the best known among the carotenoids due to many years of scientific study and publicity. It is a "pro-vitamin A carotenoid." Another way to say this is that it "has vitamin A activity." There are some other carotenoids that the human body can convert to vitamin A, but beta carotene is the primary one. Taking natural beta carotene in food is the best way to fulfill your Vitamin A needs; the body only converts as much beta carotene to Vitamin A as it needs, but at the same time beta carotene has a host of other benefits in human nutrition. First and foremost, countless studies have proven that beta-carotene has cancer-preventive qualities.

Besides beta carotene, there are a few other carotenoids that are better known than Astaxanthin. Other famous carotenoids are lutein and lycopene. Lutein has gained fame in the last decade as a nutrient for eye health; lycopene has been marketed as a preventative nutrient for prostate cancer. Both are wonderful compounds, but neither has the antioxidant and anti-inflammatory strength of Astaxanthin, nor do they have the multitude of health benefits for humans and animals.

As we move down the list of carotenoids, we notice that, although there are over 700 different carotenoids, most are not exactly household names. Some people have heard of zeaxanthin, another excellent carotenoid being marketed primarily for eye health, but how many of us have heard of echinone, gamma carotene or fucoxanthin? Not many, although the more scientists study carotenoids, the more different names you're probably going to hear. That's because many carotenoids are wonderful nutrients that can help us to live better (due to their functional properties) and live longer (due to their antioxidant and anti-inflammatory properties). And Natural Astaxanthin is the best of the bunch, although as time passes researchers may find that other carotenoids hold great promise for human health as well.

What is Astaxanthin?

Have you ever seen a bird bath in summer that has dried up? Sometimes you'll see a reddish color where the standing water has evaporated. The red you're seeing is Natural Astaxanthin. What has happened is that some green algae (perhaps the one that commercial growers of Natural Astaxanthin use which is called Haematococcus Pluvialis) have suffered stress. The stress is due to a combination of things: Lack of food, an absence of water, intense sunlight and

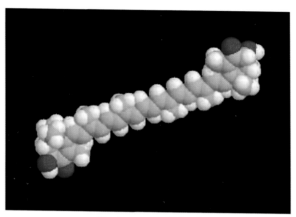

The Astaxanthin Molecule

heat, or even bitter cold. As a result of this stress, the algae's cells have hyperaccumulated the red pigment Astaxanthin. They do this as a survival mechanism— the Astaxanthin serves as a "force-field" to protect the algae from lack of nutrition and/or intense sunlight. It's an absolutely amazing fact, but due to the protective properties of Astaxanthin, these algae can stay dormant for more than forty years without food or water, suffering in the summer sun or in the winter cold; yet when conditions are appropriate and there is food and water and no extreme weather, the algae will go back into their green, motile stage.

Astaxanthin can be found in plants and animals throughout the world. It is most prevalent in algae and phytoplankton, but it also can be found in a limited number of fungi and bacteria. Because organisms like many Astaxanthin-containing algae and plankton are the base of the food chain, Astaxanthin can be found in many animals as well. Any sea animal that has a reddish or pinkish color contains Natural Astaxanthin. For example, you can find Astaxanthin in salmon, trout, lobster, shrimp and crab. These animals eat krill and other organisms that ingest Astaxanthin-containing algae and plankton as a major part of their diets. And since lots of different animals such as birds, bears and even humans eat these sea animals, you can find Astaxanthin in all sorts of places.

As we mentioned before, the animals that have the highest concentration of Astaxanthin are salmon, where it concentrates in their muscles and makes them the endurance heroes of the animal world. Can you imagine what salmon would look like if they didn't have any Astaxanthin? Not only wouldn't they be able to swim up rivers and waterfalls for days on end, but they'd also look pale and worn out.

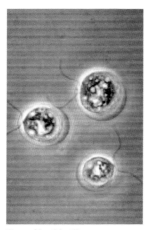

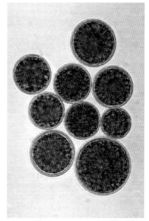

Happy, healthy Haematococcus cells in their motile, green stage.

Dormant Haematococcus cells after stress: Astaxanthin serves as a "protective force-field," enabling them to live for over forty years exposed to the elements and with no food or water.

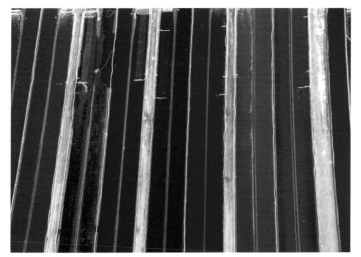

Overhead view of Haematococcus ponds in Kona, Hawaii. Similar to leaves changing colors in autumn, Haematococcus Pluvialis microalgae turn from green to red as they hyperaccumulate Astaxanthin.

9

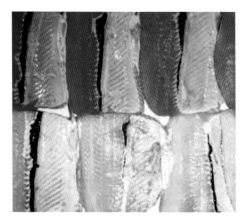

Healthy salmon fillets with plenty of Natural Astaxanthin

Sickly salmon fillets without enough Astaxanthin.

So, you see just how important Astaxanthin is for salmon. While people are not going to look all pale and sickly if they don't eat Astaxanthin in their diets, it sure can help you to look healthier and younger, and to lead a healthier, longer life.

CHAPTER 2

World's Strongest Antioxidant

Many supplements and even foods claim to be antioxidants, but only one can be the world's strongest. And Natural Astaxanthin's claim to being the "World's Strongest Natural Antioxidant" is really where it all starts: Most of Natural Astaxanthin's health benefits are in some way related to its supreme antioxidant power. In fact, the companies pioneering the use of Astaxanthin as a dietary supplement in the 1990's began promoting it as a powerful antioxidant before its other benefits were even known. Imagine how surprised they were to hear people saying that their antioxidant was taking care of their arthritis pains, giving them newfound strength and endurance, preventing them from getting colds and flu, allowing them to stay in the sun longer without burning and all sorts of other amazing results. These testimonials from early users along with increased research in the laboratory led to dozens of human clinical trials demonstrating Astaxanthin's many different applications in human nutrition. And more experiments and clinical trials are happening every year as the scientific community discovers just how great a product Natural Astaxanthin is.

Natural Astaxanthin has proven to be the strongest natural antioxidant in two separate tests. We'll study Natural Astaxanthin's incredible antioxidant ability later in this chapter, but first, let's look at what oxidation is, how antioxidants work, and why they're so important to us.

Oxygen is essential for human life. Without oxygen we would be dead in a matter of minutes. It seems strange that something that is a vital part of every breath we take can also be harmful. Yet it can. For example, oxygen is present throughout our bodies, yet if it

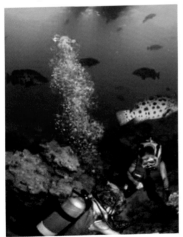

Oxygen is necessary, but can also be dangerous. Pure oxygen can actually kill a scuba diver.

11

is injected into a vein it can kill us. And pure oxygen breathed when scuba diving can also kill us.

On a cellular level, oxygen can hurt us too. Oxygen is an extremely reactive compound; during metabolism, it can combine with complex molecules to make reactive intermediate compounds which can be very destructive. The fact that oxygen is essential for aerobic organisms' life (including humans), yet is so reactive that it can be very destructive has been called the "the paradox of aerobic life" (Davies, K, 1995 and Dore, J 2003).

Free Radicals

In the body, free radicals are produced when oxygen combines with complex metabolic molecules. Free radicals are highly unstable molecules ready to react with anything they can. When they react, the result is called "oxidation." Once the oxidation process begins, it can produce a chain reaction that generates more free radicals.

Oxidation in the human body is the same thing that happens to metal when it rusts. The rusting or oxidation can destroy a strong piece of metal in just a few years. By painting the metal or putting on a rust-inhibiting product you can prevent rusting. This is the same thing that antioxidants are doing to the "rusting" in our bodies—preventing oxidation and keeping them strong. Like the rust inhibiting product which prevents the metal's cells from oxidizing and degrading, antioxidants prevent our body's cells from oxidizing and degrading. Fortunately for our bodies (and our health), antioxidants are capable of joining with oxidizing free radicals, thus rendering them harmless.

There is a very easy and interesting experiment you can do in your home that shows what oxidation is all about: Take an apple and cut it in half. Now take a lemon and cut it in half and drip the lemon juice on one half of the apple. Drip it all over the cut side of the apple, and leave the other apple half as is with no lemon juice. Keep the two halves at room temperature for an hour or two, then look at both halves: The half with the lemon juice will look pretty much the same as it did when it was cut; the half without the lemon juice will probably be turning brown and "going bad." If you leave them out longer, the difference will become more pronounced. This is oxidation and antioxidant protection happening before your eyes. The unprotected half is oxidizing quickly. The half with lemon juice is oxidizing very slowly or not at all because of the antioxidants present in the lemon juice. Lemons have Vitamin C and citrus bioflavonoids.

Although these antioxidants are nowhere nearly as strong as Natural Astaxanthin, they are strong enough to protect an apple from rotting before your eyes.

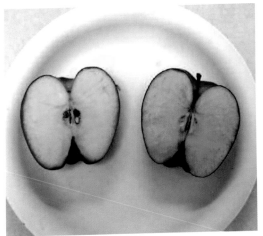

*Apple protected by antioxi-
dants Vitamin C and citrus
bioflavoids in lemon juice*   *Unprotected apple
after oxidation*

What's happening to the apple is what can happen inside our bodies if free radicals are allowed to take control. Oxidation and free radical damage show up in our bodies both externally and internally. Externally, they cause our skin to age—lines, wrinkles and dry skin—and can even cause skin cancer. Loss of muscle tone is another result of free radical damage that can actually be seen as we age.

Internally, free radicals damage tissue and can adversely affect our body's immune system. They weaken and can destroy cells and the DNA in the cells. Scientists believe that DNA damage is a major component of the aging process. DNA is an amazing substance that tells cells when to divide, how to make enzymes and other proteins, and how to direct all the other cellular activities. If DNA is damaged, cells cease to function normally, causing a host of potential problems and diseases. Damaged DNA can be repaired, but occasionally the repair job is defective—in the worst case, a cancerous cell line can begin. Our body's immune system sometimes detects and eliminates cancerous cell lines, but of course, it is better to avoid this last line of defense and prevent the DNA damage in the first place. Antioxidants can help neutralize free radicals and steer us

13

clear of cell damage before it even begins to occur.

Because of their ability to eliminate free radicals, antioxidants can help slow the aging process. Some amazing research was done recently at the University of Washington. Mice were genetically engineered to load an antioxidant into the mitochondria of the cells. These mice lived 20% longer than the control group and had less heart disease and cataracts! "In short, they were biologically younger. It's the best proof yet that antioxidants can slow aging" (Carper, J, 2005).

Causes of Free Radical Production

There are many different causes of free radical production. Normal body processes such as digestion and breathing produce small quantities of free radicals. The functioning of our immune system also produces free radicals. Exercise causes free radicals to be produced too. These are all normal things that people do every day, and our bodies were designed to handle the free radicals produced without taking antioxidant supplements in two ways: First of all, our bodies produce their own antioxidants to neutralize this normal level of free radical generation. For instance, enzymes produced by the body such as superoxide dismutase are effective in eliminating free radical molecules. Some can quench singlet oxygen which is a very unstable form of oxygen that causes oxidative damage.

The second way our bodies neutralize free radicals is through dietary antioxidants in the foods we eat. Every time you eat an orange you are eating a few different antioxidants such as Vitamin C and citrus bioflavonoids. Similarly, when you eat some green leafy vegetables you are probably getting a few different, more powerful antioxidant carotenoids like beta carotene and lutein.

The problem with self-produced antioxidants like superoxide dismutase and dietary antioxidants like Vitamin C and beta carotene is that we don't get enough of them to handle all the free radicals in our bodies. This is due to diets that do not have enough fruits and vegetables, but there is another, more important reason: Our bodies now produce and absorb more free radicals than our ancestors due to the lifestyles we lead and the world we now live in.

Large amounts of free radicals are produced when we are under stress. There is no doubt that humans in the 21st century are much more subject to stress than humans were 100 or more years ago. Hectic, busy lifestyles common today account for levels of free radical production that were not known to our grandparents. Consequently, the amount of antioxidants produced by our own bodies added to the amount of antioxidants consumed even in a healthy diet are not enough to ward off the ravages of stress-caused free radicals in most people today. This is one of the reasons most nutrition experts recommend that we supplement our diets with antioxidants—as added protection for today's busy lifestyles.

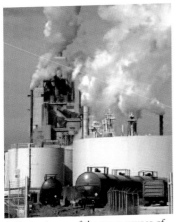

Pollution is one of the many causes of increased oxidation and free radical damage for humans living in today's world.

Another cause of increased levels of free radicals in humans living today is the high quantity of contaminants present today that didn't exist a few generations ago. Huge quantities of free radicals are present in different pollutants like chemicals, car exhaust, smoke and even burnt or barbecued food. Processed foods with all sorts of engineered compounds in unnatural forms are another source of free radicals relatively new to humans.

Exposure to sunlight is another increasing source of free radical formation to contend with in modern life. The sun's rays can cause high levels of free radicals in the skin that can lead to skin cancers. This is a huge concern nowadays as we are exposed to higher levels of ultraviolet rays due to polluting gases diminishing the ozone layer. Levels of skin cancer including the deadly melanoma are rising exponentially, and this can be linked directly to free radicals caused by increased UV exposure (Ames and Shigenaga 1992, 1993; Harman 1981; Esterbauer et al., 1992). The sun's rays can quickly destroy cells, but antioxidants can do a great deal to protect cells. With the increase in UV levels, pollutants in the environment and the high levels of stress in modern life, it's easy to see why we can't rely on our own body's antioxidant production to save us any more. Not even the best diets have enough antioxidants present to protect us from today's onslaught of free radicals and singlet oxygen, so supplementing with strong antioxidants is critical to maintaining good health.

Another cause of increased free radical production common today is found in athletes as well as ordinary citizens who participate in demanding sports. The body produces large quantities of free radicals during strenuous exercise or even

15

during hard physical work. This is caused by the body burning more fuel for energy (Dekkers, 1996; Witt, 1992; Goldfarb, 1999). Anyone who is exercising or doing hard physical work, especially when outdoors in the sun, is producing levels of free radicals that necessitate antioxidant supplementation. Many athletes swear that they can actually feel the difference when they take strong antioxidant supplements, resulting in better, longer workouts, faster recoveries and better performance. We'll study this phenomenon in more detail later.

Antioxidants: A Daily Regimen

There are many different types of antioxidants. Enzymes can be antioxidants, vitamins can be antioxidants and phytonutrients such as carotenoids can be antioxidants to name just a few. Recent studies have shown that many common foods have some antioxidant abilities, and marketers are starting to mention this in advertising and on product labels as a selling point. In just the last few years foods such as blueberries, spinach and oranges have been marketed as antioxidants. But we're also hearing that coffee, tea and even beer are also antioxidants. Who should we believe?

To be honest, all of these products probably have some antioxidant properties. But there are two critical points to consider when judging antioxidant consumption and deciding what you should eat and what supplements you should take: First is antioxidant strength. In order to derive benefits from free radical elimination, for example, you can eat lots and lots of a food that has a low level of antioxidant activity, or you can take a concentrated supplement in pill form that has a very high level of antioxidant activity.

The second point to consider somewhat contradicts the first: Antioxidants are best taken with an assortment of other antioxidants. Antioxidants work together and can actually be synergistic: Two or three antioxidants can have a combined effect greater than the sum of the individual antioxidants. Here is where eating a varied diet with a minimum of five to nine servings of fruits and vegetables comes into play. You cannot get the variety of antioxidants in their natural states that exist in nine servings of produce from a bottle. But what you can and should do to ensure proper antioxidant protection is:

- Eat a good diet each day with lots of fresh fruits and vegetables (preferably nine servings!)
- Take a high quality multivitamin

· Take a green food supplement like Spirulina
· Take a powerful antioxidant like Natural Astaxanthin

By following this diet and supplement regimen, you'll get a great diversity of antioxidants from the produce with all its live enzymes and phytonutrients. You'll get good amounts of vitamin antioxidants such as natural Vitamin E and C as well as commonly missed antioxidants like selenium from a good multivitamin. You'll cover lots of potentially missed antioxidants, vitamins, enzymes and phytonutrients from a good green food supplement like Spirulina. And last but not least, you'll get powerful, concentrated free radical elimination and singlet oxygen quenching from Natural Astaxanthin.

Nature's Ultimate Antioxidant: Astaxanthin!

Astaxanthin has been shown in two different in-vitro experiments to be the strongest natural antioxidant known to science. There are many different ways to measure antioxidant strength. One popular measurement today is called Oxygen Radical Absorbance Capacity (ORAC, as developed by Brunswick Labs, Norton, Massachusetts, USA). According to Brunswick Labs, the ORAC test is not a good measurement for oil soluble carotenoids like Astaxanthin, so Natural Astaxanthin was examined by two alternative procedures. In the two antioxidant tests that we've seen to date, Astaxanthin left all competitors far behind.

In the first experiment on page 18, Astaxanthin yielded an antioxidant strength 550 times stronger than Vitamin E in singlet oxygen quenching (Shimidzu et al, 1996). Vitamin E has been touted to be a strong antioxidant both internally and in topical uses in cosmetics; yet Astaxanthin's antioxidant strength completely dwarfed Vitamin E!

It's also very interesting to note Astaxanthin's relationship to the closely related carotenoid beta carotene. Beta carotene is the most widely researched carotenoid and is certainly a wonderful compound with many health benefits. It is a carotenoid with Vitamin A activity—it is converted into Vitamin A in the human body as needed. As we examined in the first chapter, Astaxanthin is very similar chemically to beta carotene. Yet Astaxanthin was 11 times stronger than beta carotene in singlet oxygen quenching!

Lutein has become a very well known product over the last ten years. It is also a carotenoid like beta carotene and Astaxanthin. Lutein has been marketed as a great product for eye health (although we'll discuss in a later chapter evi-

17

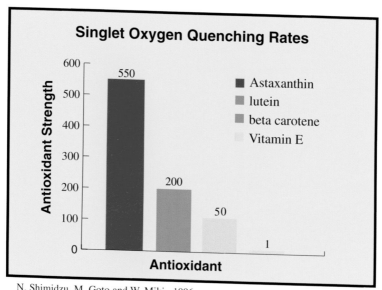

N. Shimidzu, M. Goto and W. Miki. 1996

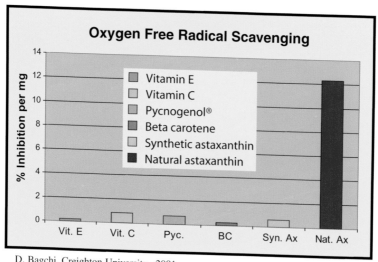

D. Bagchi, Creighton University. 2001

dence that Astaxanthin may in fact be better for eye health than lutein). As an antioxidant targeting harmful singlet oxygen, Astaxanthin proved to be almost three times stronger than lutein.

The second study was done at Creighton University; it measured Natural Astaxanthin (as BioAstin® from Cyanotech Corporation) against Vitamin E, Vitamin C, Pycnogenol®, Beta Carotene and other antioxidants (including synthetic astaxanthin) as a free radical scavenger. In this experiment Natural Astaxanthin ranged from a minimum of 14 times stronger to over 60 times stronger than all the other antioxidants! (Bagchi, 2001). The breakdown is as follows:

Natural Astaxanthin as BioAstin® from Cyanotech Corp.	14.3 times stronger than Vitamin E
	17.9 times stronger than Pycnogenol®
	20.9 times stronger than Synthetic Astaxanthin
	53.7 times stronger than Beta Carotene
	64.9 times stronger than Vitamin C

It is remarkable to note how different types of antioxidant testing can yield drastically different results. For example, in the first test measuring singlet oxygen quenching, Astaxanthin proved to be 550 times stronger than Vitamin E. In this test measuring free radical scavenging, Astaxanthin was only 14.3 times stronger than Vitamin E. This is why it can be misleading to rely on a single test to measure antioxidant strength: Results can vary dramatically. It is better to look for patterns. The pattern that emerges after examining results from these two extremely different tests as well as other research on antioxidants is that Astaxanthin is the most powerful natural antioxidant of all.

Natural versus Synthetic Astaxanthin

A fascinating point to consider is how Natural Astaxanthin performed in the free radical scavenging antioxidant test versus Synthetic Astaxanthin. Synthetic Astaxanthin is produced by a few huge chemical companies in the laboratory from petrochemicals. Although it has the same exact chemical formula as Natural Astaxanthin, it is actually a different molecule—the shape of the molecule is different, plus in its natural state, Astaxanthin is always paired with fatty acids attached to the end of the Astaxanthin molecule. This results in an "esterified" molecule, and makes Natural Astaxanthin far superior to Synthetic Astaxanthin as an antioxidant and in many other ways, which we'll explore later.

Another critical difference is that the Natural Astaxanthin tested (BioAstin® from Cyanotech Corporation in Hawaii) is extracted from Haematococcus Pluvialis microalgae. When the microalgae hyperaccumulates Astaxanthin as a survival mechanism due to environmental stress, it also produces small quantities of other supporting carotenoids. The resulting complex is broken down as follows:

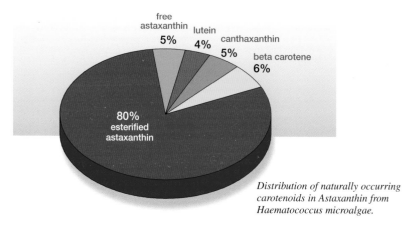

Distribution of naturally occurring carotenoids in Astaxanthin from Haematococcus microalgae.

The additional carotenoids beta carotene, canthaxanthin and lutein work in synergy to make Natural Astaxanthin a more effective antioxidant than Synthetic Astaxanthin. At the same time, they lead to much more efficacy in treating various health conditions and ensuring Natural Astaxanthin's many health benefits. We'll discuss the difference between Natural Astaxanthin and synthetic Astaxanthin in more detail in Chapter 9.

Antioxidant for the Brain, Eyes and Central Nervous System

Many antioxidants and even carotenoids that are closely related to Natural Astaxanthin cannot cross the blood-brain barrier and get into the brain, the eyes and the central nervous system. Even beta carotene, the most well known of all carotenoids cannot do this. Neither can some other well known carotenoids such as lycopene. But Astaxanthin can! This is vital for antioxidants because scientists currently theorize that diseases and injuries of the eye and central nervous system are caused by the increased generation and presence of singlet oxygen and other free radicals (superoxide, hydroxyl, hydrogen peroxide, etc.) or by decreased free radical removal ability. Such diseases include age-related macular degeneration (the leading cause of blindness in the United States), retinal arterial and venous occlusion, glaucoma, diabetic retinopathy and injuries resulting from trauma and inflammation. An antioxidant that can reach the inner eye by crossing the blood-brain and blood-retinal barriers would protect the eye from these damaging conditions.

Although Astaxanthin is not normally found in the eye, Dr. Mark Tso was the first to prove that Astaxanthin could cross the blood-brain and blood-retinal barriers by feeding Astaxanthin to rats and finding it in their eyes. He then proved it protected the eye from light-induced damage, photoreceptor cell damage, ganglion cell damage, neuronal damage and inflammatory damage (Tso, et al, 1996). Astaxanthin may be the absolute best protection for the eyes among any supplements, although researchers are just beginning to find out about this now.

Never a "Pro-Oxidant"

There is a potential for some wonderful antioxidants, under certain conditions, to become "pro-oxidants" and actually have a negative effect by causing oxidation in the body. Some of the better-known carotenoid antioxidants that can become pro-oxidants are beta carotene, lycopene and zeaxanthin (Martin, et al, 1999). Even such familiar antioxidants as vitamin C, vitamin E and zinc can become pro-oxidants. This is another important factor separating Astaxanthin from other antioxidants—it never becomes a pro-oxidant (Beutner, et al, 2000). This is one more reason that Astaxanthin is clearly a superior antioxidant to others.

A famous study of beta carotene on smokers was done in Finland in the 1990's. In this study, it was found that smokers who took synthetic beta carotene supplements actually had a higher incidence of cancer than those taking a placebo. The challenge with beta-carotene is that it relies on other antioxidants, specifically vitamin C, to properly protect cells from free radicals. (Try to think of a free radical as a hot potato that needs to be passed from one antioxidant to another until it cools off.)

The people in this study were very heavy smokers (three packs per day)

21

and not representative of the general population. In addition, the increase in the incidence of cancer was so small as to not be statistically significant; but in any event, it was very unusual to think that taking synthetic beta carotene might increase the risk of cancer, particularly after over two hundred previous studies of diet and cancer indicated that diets rich in foods containing beta carotene were correlated with a lower incidence of cancer. (Upon further review of this Finnish study, it was found that the subjects in the study that had eaten the most dietary natural beta carotene as compared to taking synthetic supplemental beta carotene also had the lowest incidence of cancer, as would be expected from previous studies.) (Malila, et al, 2006)

So what was going on? Two things: First, it should be noted that diets containing high levels of foods rich in beta-carotene also contain large amounts of other naturally occurring carotenoids and antioxidants, including forms of natural beta carotene not found in the synthetic supplement. So the "hot potato" can be passed from antioxidant to antioxidant until it is neutralized. Secondly, this study was with heavy smokers, who tend to be depleted in Vitamin C. Without vitamin C, beta carotene can catch the destructive energy of a free radical and itself become a damaging molecule. In this situation, beta carotene has entered into a "pro-oxidant" state. If Vitamin C is available, this pro-oxidant state will quickly be converted back to an antioxidant state without damage to cells.

Fortunately, slight differences in the molecular constituents of Astaxanthin have the effect of preventing a pro-oxidant state. This means that, unlike beta carotene, lycopene, zeaxanthin and Vitamins C and E, Astaxanthin never becomes a pro-oxidant and thus can never be harmful for anyone, including smokers or other people that might have low levels of Vitamin C.

CHAPTER 3

Safe, Natural Anti-Inflammatory

Anti-inflammatories have gotten a bad reputation. There's aspirin which can cause stomach bleeding. Then there's acetaminophen (Tylenol®) which can cause liver damage. Then came along the strong Cox-2 inhibitors such as Vioxx® and Celebrex®. Well, it turns out that these can potentially cause heart problems. The fact is that most anti-inflammatories have a potential for dangerous side effects. The American Journal of Medicine reported that non-steroidal anti-inflammatory drugs (NSAID's) contribute to roughly 16,500 deaths and more than 100,000 hospitalizations each year! (Singh, G, 1998). The New England Journal of Medicine compared the number of deaths from NSAID's as being similar to the number of deaths from AIDS (Wolf, et al, 1999). Many people with arthritis will try glucosamine and chondroitin. But these products are proving to help only a fraction of the people who try them. A large scale study in which subjects took either 1500 mg of glucosamine sulfate alone, 1200 mg of chondroitin alone or a combination of both showed no statistically significant differences from the placebo group. It should be noted that a subgroup of patients with mod-

Over 80% of Arthritis Sufferers Improve with Astaxanthin!

A health questionnaire of 247 Astaxanthin users showed that "Over 80% of those reporting back pain and symptoms from osteoarthritis or rheumatoid arthritis reported an improvement from Astaxanthin supplementation. Astaxanthin supplementation was also reported to improve symptoms of asthma and enlarged prostate. All of these conditions have an inflammation component which is closely tied to oxidative damage." *(Guerin, et al, 2002)*

erate to severe pain resulted in a majority experiencing a reduction in pain by at least 20%, but overall the results add to a contradictory body of evidence on the effectiveness of glucosamine and chondroitin (Clegg, et al, 2006). What's a person with arthritis, tendonitis or just good old-fashioned aches and pains to do? They should try Natural Astaxanthin.

We should give a word of warning here: Astaxanthin may not work as strongly or certainly not as quickly as Vioxx, but fortunately it's a safe, natural alternative. Most people will not see benefits in pain relief or increased strength and mobility for two to four weeks after taking Astaxanthin, and to be honest, as many as 25% of people may have reduced or even negligible results. This is the nature of natural remedies—they aren't as concentrated as prescription medications, so they won't work overnight. And due to the different metabolisms and the different types of bodies people have, they may not work perfectly for everyone. In different clinical studies on inflammatory conditions, Natural Astaxanthin has been shown to be very effective for the majority of people, but there are some who don't get the desired results. But even with prescription drugs such as Vioxx and Celebrex and over-the-counter products such as aspirin and Tylenol, there are also people who don't get results, and with these products there are dangerous side effects. Natural Astaxanthin, on the other hand, has never been shown to have any negative side effect or contraindication. The only potential effect from people taking megadosis far above the recommended 4 – 12 mg per day may be a slight orange color in the palms of the hands and soles of the feet. This is due to the pigment in Astaxanthin depositing in the skin, and as we'll see later, this is a good thing since it's what allows Astaxanthin to work as an internal sunscreen.

What Exactly is Inflammation?

Inflammation is essential for our survival. It is our bodies' immune response to fight infection and repair damaged tissues. It is a complex physical and biochemical process. Basically, inflammation is the healing process that is triggered when there is something wrong with our bodies. If an unwanted bacteria or virus attacks us, our inflammatory system kicks in and starts to fight against it. If we sprain an ankle, again, our inflammatory system begins to work to repair the damaged tissues. Without an inflammatory system, we would soon be dead.

Inflammation shows up in many different ways. For example, the swelling that occurs after we sprain our ankles is a sign of inflammation. The red knuck-

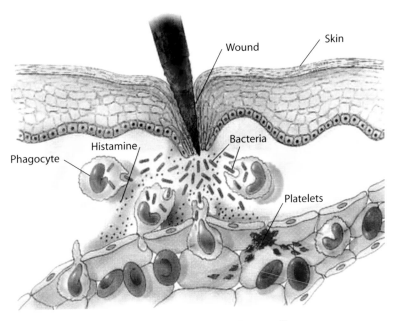

Overview of the Human Inflammatory Response System

les of a person with arthritis is another sure sign of inflammation. Even sunburn is a sign of inflammation; when the ultraviolet rays of the sun begin to damage our skin cells, our inflammatory systems turn on and our skin turns red.

An in-depth discussion of the human inflammatory response is beyond the scope of this book; it is an extremely complicated process. The illustration above gives a broad overview of the process. Most of our tissues have cells in them called "mast cells." Mast cells are the key initiators of inflammation. They release many potent inflammation mediators. These mediators either attract white blood cells, or activate cells that have been attracted to produce additional mediators.

There are many different inflammation mediators. Among those that are known and understood are histamine, tumor necrosis factor-alpha, reactive oxygen species such as nitric oxide and hydrogen peroxide, interleukins and prostaglandins. Prostaglandins are produced from arachidonic acid and by cyclooxygenases, the COX-1 and COX-2 enzymes. As we mentioned before, the prescription anti-inflammatories Vioxx and Celebrex are very strong, specific COX-2 inhibitors. On the other hand, aspirin is a non-specific COX inhibitor in that it controls both the COX-1 and COX-2 enzymes. Astaxanthin is very different from these other products in that it has an effect on many different mediators, but in a gentler, less concentrated manner. This is how Astaxanthin can be an effective anti-inflammatory without any negative side effects.

Mechanism of Action

Due to the multitude of ways in which Astaxanthin combats inflammation, it is a very special anti-inflammatory indeed. Both in-vitro and in-vivo research has been done to uncover Astaxanthin's mechanism of action. This mechanism has been further demonstrated in several double blind, placebo controlled human clinical trials on various inflammatory conditions.

Astaxanthin's anti-inflammatory properties are closely related to its powerful antioxidant activity. Many antioxidants exhibit an anti-inflammatory effect as well. To a certain extent, because Astaxanthin is the most powerful natural antioxidant, it is also a very effective anti-inflammatory.

Astaxanthin works to suppress different inflammatory mediators. Among these mediators are tumor necrosis factor alpha (TNF-a), prostaglandin E-2 (PGE-2), interleukin 1B (IL-1b) and nitric oxide (NO). In one experiment done with mice and also in-vitro, Astaxanthin was shown to suppress TNF-a, PGE-2, IL-1b, NO as well as the Cox-2 enzyme and nuclear factor kappa-B (Lee, et al, 2003).

Another study done the same year was led by a researcher from Japan's Hokkaido University Graduate School of Medicine. Here, the researchers found similar results: Astaxanthin was shown in vitro to decrease the production of NO, PGE-2 and TNF-a. This study also looked at Astaxanthin's anti-inflammatory effect in the eyes of rats. The researchers induced uveitis (inflammation of the inner eye including the iris) and found that Astaxanthin had a "dose dependent ocular anti-inflammatory effect, by the suppression of NO, PGE-2 and TNF-a production, through directly blocking nitric oxide synthase enzyme activity" (Ohgami, et al, 2003). Basically, this study proved that Astaxanthin reduces inflammation of the eye, the root cause of many different vision ailments, and clearly demonstrated exactly how it does this.

The graphs on pages 27 and 28 visually depict how Astaxanthin works to combat inflammation through multiple pathways.

COMBINED RESULTS FROM INFLAMMATORY MECHANISM RESEARCH

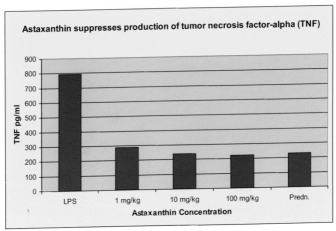

TUMER NECROSIS FACTOR

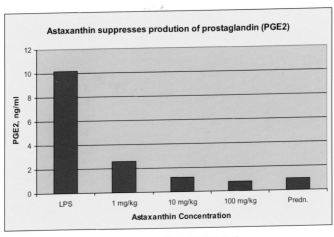

PROSTAGLANDIN E-2

Measurement of the anti-inflammatory action of Astaxanthin in lipopolysaccharide (LPS) induced inflammation in rats, as measured by tumor necrosis factor and prostaglandin E-2, and compared with the anti-inflammatory drug prednisolone (Ohgami, et al, 2003).

27

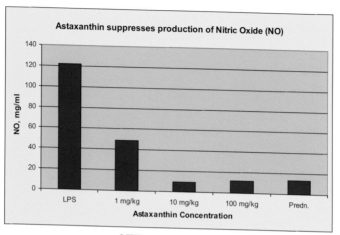

NITRIC OXIDE

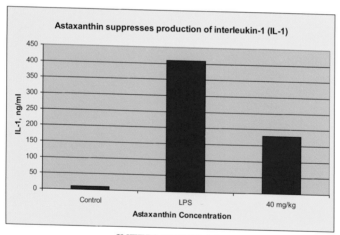

INTERLEUKIN 1-B

The top graph shows the measurement of the anti-inflammatory action of Astaxanthin in lipopolysaccharide (LPS) induced inflammation in rats as measured by nitric oxide levels, and compared with the anti-inflammatory drug prednisolone (Ohgami, et al, 2003). The bottom graph shows the measurement of anti-inflammatory action of Astaxanthin in LPS induced inflammation in mice as measured by interleukin 1-B (Lee, et al, 2003).

Another pathway in which Astaxanthin combats inflammation is through inhibition of the cyclooxygenase enzymes (Cox-1 and Cox-2). As we mentioned before, Vioxx and Celebrex work as intense Cox-2 inhibitors. The concentrated way in which they work leads to undesired side effects, such as the heart problems that were publicized in 2004. Lee, et al, demonstrated that Astaxanthin has a Cox-2 inhibitory effect. But Cyanotech Corporation, a commercial producer of Natural Astaxanthin from microalgae (trademarked as BioAstin®) wanted a better understanding of this critical matter. They wanted to demonstrate that the Cox-2 effect of Natural Astaxanthin is very different and much less intense than that of prescription medications. Cyanotech contracted a very well respected independent laboratory to analyze the drug Celecoxib (distributed as Celebrex®) in relation to Natural Astaxanthin (distributed as BioAstin®). The laboratory found that Celecoxib was over 300 times stronger in Cox-2 inhibition than Natural Astaxanthin. However, in Cox-1 inhibition, the two were much closer in strength: Celecoxib was only 4.4 times stronger. Of course, the ratio of Cox-2 to Cox-1 inhibition for each product was also very different: For Celecoxib the ratio was 78.5, while for Natural Astaxanthin it was only 1.1. This illustrates that Cox-2 and Cox-1 inhibition by Natural Astaxanthin is almost the same (Brunswick Laboratories, 2004). More research would have to be done to better understand the full impact of this enormous difference, but the logical conclusion is that Celebrex and Vioxx work faster because they are extremely focused in their Cox-2 inhibition, but this leads to dangerous side effects. Contrarily, Natural Astaxanthin works slower but exhibits no side effects. "While [anti-inflammatory] drugs usually block a single target molecule and reduce its activity dramatically, natural anti-inflammatories gently tweak a broader range of inflammatory compounds. You'll get greater safety and efficacy reducing five inflammatory mediators by 30 percent than by reducing one by 100%" (Cole, G, 2005). After analyzing all the pluses and minuses of aspirin, acetaminophen, prescription anti-inflammatories and Natural Astaxanthin, it becomes very clear that Natural Astaxanthin is the only smart choice — it's safe, and it works for a high percentage of people.

"Silent" Inflammation and C-Reactive Protein

While sporadic inflammation is a normal and healthy process, prolonged inflammation can be devastating. Prolonged inflammation can lead to tissue damage and many serious diseases. Recently, scientists have been studying prolonged, low level inflammation that many people experience without even knowing it. This is called systemic or "silent" inflammation. "A decade ago, researchers were blaming oxidative damage for everything from cancer to heart disease. Now, chronic, low-grade inflammation is seizing the spotlight. 'Inflammation is the evil twin of oxidation,' says neuroscientist James Joseph of Tufts University. 'Where you find one, you find the other.' That would include not only such obvious inflammatory conditions as asthma and rheumatoid arthritis, but also ailments never previously associated with inflammation—such as atherosclerosis, Alzheimer's disease, colon cancer and diabetes" (Underwood, A, 2005).

The number of diseases linked to silent inflammation is staggering: Heart disease, stroke, cancer, diabetes, Alzheimer's, Parkinson's, asthma, rheumatoid arthritis, ulcers, irritable bowel syndrome and more. We can feel perfectly healthy while silent inflammation slowly ravages our bodies, creating the diseases that will ultimately kill us.

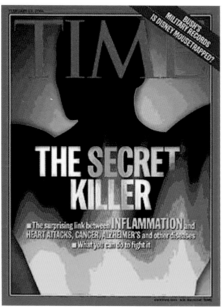

February, 2004 front cover story on "silent" inflammation, Time Magazine

Silent inflammation has become such a hot topic that the mainstream media has begun to focus on it. While we used to constantly hear about oxidation and free radicals in the media during the 1990's, it seems that with the new millennium, the buzz-word of the day is inflammation. The truth of the matter is that both are interrelated, and it is extremely important to combat both.

Long time health advocate, Dr. Barry Sears, is the President of the Inflammation Research Foundation. Dr. Sears wrote an outstanding article recently on "silent inflammation." Dr Sears said, "What if there was a condition that threatened to destroy the entire US healthcare system in a very short time? Every politician would be making speeches about it. There would be a mobilization of the entire medical establishment to combat it…Unfortunately, such a condition does exist and no one seems concerned about it. This condition is 'silent inflammation'…Silent inflammation is different from classical inflammation in that it is below the threshold of perceived pain. As a result, no action is taken to stop it, and it lingers for years, if not decades, causing continued insults on the heart, the immune system and the brain." Dr. Sears points out that Americans have the highest levels of silent inflammation in the world with over 75% of people afflicted. He says that there is no drug that can reverse silent inflammation, "but there are anti-inflammatory diets and anti-inflammatory dietary supplements that can" (Sears, B, 2005).

The most common test for silent inflammation is a measurement of blood levels of a substance called C-reactive protein (CRP). In 2003, a panel of experts convened by the American Heart Association and the Center for Disease Control and Prevention recommended the CRP blood test as a way of assessing heart disease risk. Researchers from leading institutions such as Harvard among many others have declared that CRP is a more reliable indicator of heart disease risk than cholesterol testing. CRP is produced in the liver and in the coronary arteries, and is then released into the bloodstream when the body is fighting inflammation. It is a marker for inflammatory activity, but it does not cause inflammation (Perry, S, 2006).

In 2006, a human clinical study analyzed the effects of Natural Astaxanthin on blood CRP levels. The study was conducted at the Health Research and Studies Center in California, an independent research company that specializes in nutraceutical clinical work. The research was headed by Gene Spiller, PhD. Dr. Spiller had done previous work with Natural Astaxanthin, and in fact had focused on Natural Astaxanthin's effects on various inflammatory conditions. This study was done with a relatively small sample size, with twenty five subjects completing the full course. The study lasted for eight weeks. Sixteen subjects received Natural Astaxanthin and nine received a placebo. Blood CRP levels were measured before the subjects began the supplement regimen, and again at the end of the study. The results were extremely promising: On average, the treatment group experienced a 20.7% reduction in CRP levels in just eight weeks, while the placebo group saw an increase in their levels (Spiller, et al, 2006a).

Another study on the effects of Natural Astaxanthin on CRP was publicized in 2006, although not published in a peer reviewed journal. This study specifically used subjects with elevated CRP levels that would put them in a high risk category. After three months in the ongoing study, 43% of the treatment group experienced enough of a reduction in their blood CRP levels to fall out of the high risk category and into the average risk group. To the contrary, all of the subjects in the placebo groups remained at high risk (Mera Pharmaceuticals, 2006). The study is continuing for a further, long-term analysis, but the results after three months are very positive: Close to half of the subjects returned their CRP levels from high risk to normal by supplementing their diets with Natural Astaxanthin!

Tennis Elbow (Tendonitis)

It appears that Astaxanthin can have a significant effect on inflammation of the tendons. A very interesting study was conducted by Dr. Spiller from the Health Research and Studies Center on patients suffering from tennis elbow. Tennis elbow is a form of tendonitis. One of the debilitating results of this condition is the decrease in grip strength and pain that is generated when gripping something in the hand. Dr. Spiller analyzed the effect of Astaxanthin supplementation on the grip strength of tennis elbow sufferers.

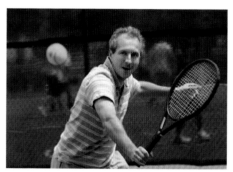

This study was comprised of thirty three subjects who completed the eight week course of supplementation or placebo. Twenty one subjects received Natural Astaxanthin gelcaps, while twelve received a placebo. Grip strength was measured at the beginning of the eight week trial and again at the end of the trial.

After eight weeks of taking Natural Astaxanthin, the treatment group showed a remarkable average improvement in grip strength of 93%, while at the same time self-assessment of their pain level decreased. Dr. Spiller wrote, "The group receiving BioAstin® [Natural Astaxanthin] had a significant increase in grip strength measurement when compared to the group receiving the placebo...This correlation of improved grip strength measurement and BioAstin® may suggest that daily use can help alleviate pain associated with tennis elbow and increase mobility. This improve-

Tennis elbow causes loss of grip strength, pain and loss of mobility

ment may greatly improve the standard of living for those who suffer from such joint disorders" (Spiller, et al, 2006b).

Carpal Tunnel Syndrome (Repetitive Stress Injury)

Dr. Spiller and his research partner, Yael Nir, MD, had previously studied a related tendon condition known as "carpal tunnel syndrome" (CTS) in some countries, or alternatively as "repetitive stress injury" in other countries. CTS is a debilitating disease of the wrist that manifests itself in numbness, pain and in extreme cases even paralysis. There is no cure for this condition; current medical procedures are to put a splint on the wrists to immobilize it or, at the very least, restrict movement to a minimum. If the condition doesn't improve after immobilization, most often wrist surgery is recommended. Unfortunately, not all patients respond to surgery. Clearly, an alternative therapy that addresses the symptoms of CTS would be extremely beneficial.

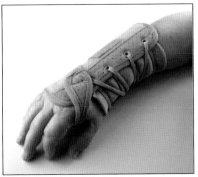

There is no cure for carpal tunnel syndrome. Conventional therapy involves splints or surgery.

The clinical trial done on CTS sufferers was done with twenty subjects, thirteen in the treatment group and seven in the placebo group over an eight week period. The participants completed a questionnaire three times during the study, at the beginning, after four weeks and again at the end, after eight weeks. Each time they answered questions on the number of times a day they experienced pain (pain rate) and the duration of their pain. The analysis of the questionnaires showed that the participants who were taking the astaxanthin-containing capsules experienced a marked decrease in daytime pain rate and duration of pain at mid-study (after 4 weeks) and an even greater decrease at the end of the study (after 8 weeks).

The result showed that the group taking Natural Astaxanthin reported a 27% reduction in daytime pain after four weeks and a 41% reduction after eight weeks. Similarly, the duration of daytime pain decreased by 21% after four weeks and 36% after eight weeks. The researchers noted that some subjects reported major changes were possible in their lifestyle after using Natural Astaxanthin (Nir

IMPROVEMENT IN CARPAL TUNNEL SUFFERERS

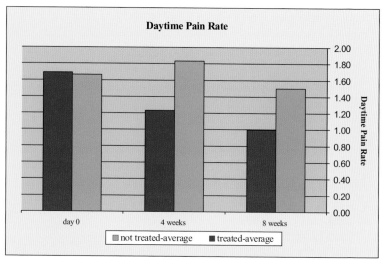

Daytime pain rate at the beginning, mid-way, and end of the study.

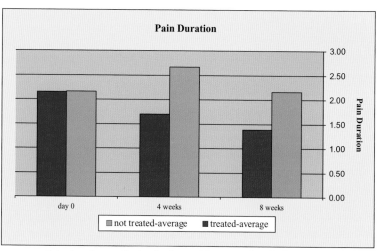

Pain duration at the beginning, mid-way, and end of the study.

and Spiller, 2002a). This study as well as extensive anecdotal evidence from carpal tunnel sufferers shows that Natural Astaxanthin may be a viable alternative to surgery.

Rheumatoid Arthritis

An extremely promising clinical trial was completed by Drs. Nir and Spiller on rheumatoid arthritis sufferers. Rheumatoid arthritis is an auto-immune disorder in which the sufferer's own immune system attacks itself. Rheumatoid

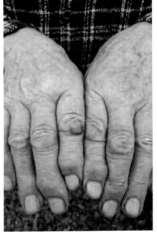

Hands Crippled by Rheumatoid Arthritis

arthritis is much more difficult to treat than osteo arthritis. It is a chronic destructive disorder that can cripple sufferers. Unfortunately, many traditional therapies are not very effective, and prescription drugs may be unsafe as well as ineffective. Alternative therapies and nutraceuticals before Natural Astaxanthin have yielded inconsistent results.

This study featured twenty one subjects, fourteen receiving Astaxanthin and seven receiving a placebo. Duration of the study was eight weeks. Pain and satisfaction with the ability to perform daily activities were measured at the beginning of the study, after four weeks, and finally after eight weeks of treatment.

The results showed a significant difference both in pain and satisfaction scores between the treatment and control groups at the end of the study. Pain scores for the treatment group decreased by approximately 10% after four weeks, and by more than 35% after eight weeks. The pain scores for the placebo group remained relatively constant. The subjects self-rated satisfaction scores with those receiving Natural Astaxanthin improving by approximately 15% after four weeks and by over 40% after eight weeks. These results were extremely significant, and the researchers concluded that "Astaxanthin-based supplements appear to be an effective addition in the treatment of rheumatoid arthritis and further studies should be carried out with a larger population" (Nir and Spiller, 2002b). Once again, Natural Astaxanthin demonstrated that it could help people suffering with serious inflammatory conditions live better, happier lives.

Joint Soreness after Exercise

Before Dr. Spiller and Dr. Nir began their extensive research on Natural Astaxanthin's anti-inflammatory properties in human clinical trials, another researcher, Andrew Fry, PhD, found positive results on an inflammatory condition in a very different group of subjects. These people were not suffering from any sort of disease or affliction.

Dr. Fry is a professor at the University of Memphis, where he serves as the Director of the Exercise Biochemistry Laboratory. Dr. Fry did a clinical trial to see how Natural Astaxanthin could help people that exercise overcome the common joint and muscle soreness that occurs in the days following their strenuous activity. He recruited twenty young men who regularly trained with weights, since this type of person would frequently experience exercise-induced joint soreness. This study ran for only three weeks, a relatively short period when considered in respect to Astaxanthin's cumulative nature as it concentrates throughout the body over time. The treatment and placebo groups were subjected to strenuous knee exercises on a resistance-training apparatus.

The placebo group experienced significant joint pain in their knees when surveyed immediately after the strenuous knee workout, and also at intervals of ten hours, twenty four hours and forty eight hours afterward. Remarkably, the young men taking Natural Astaxanthin showed no increase whatsoever in joint soreness in their knees. It appeared that Natural Astaxanthin at a moderate dose of 4 mg per day completely prevented joint pain after exercise (Fry, A, 2001).

This clinical trial is extremely significant as it shows how Natural Astaxanthin's anti-inflammatory properties can help all kinds of people—not just those who suffer from inflammatory diseases—but pretty much anyone who exercises or does strenuous work. From top athletes to weekend warriors, from homeowners working in their gardens to people crippled with rheumatoid arthritis, Natural Astaxanthin can help reduce pain and inflammation in tendons, joints and muscles. It can help control the ravages of "silent" inflammation and prevent the myriad of diseases it causes. Powerful antioxidant, safe and natural anti-inflammatory, Natural Astaxanthin is a great supplement for everyone!

CHAPTER 4

Healthy Eyes, Healthy Brain

Other carotenoids have begun to attain a certain level of fame for having beneficial properties for the eyes. There is no doubt that lutein and zeaxanthin are wonderful products to support and protect the eyes, and there is credible evidence that they can help prevent age related macular degeneration and other degenerative conditions. But due to Natural Astaxanthin's superior antioxidant and anti-inflammatory properties, indications are that it will prove to be superior to all other nutraceuticals for eye and brain health.

As we briefly discussed in Chapter 2, many antioxidants and even carotenoids that are closely related to Natural Astaxanthin cannot cross the blood-brain barrier. This means that they can't do anything to help the brain, the eyes or the central nervous system, and we all know how vital these organs are. Beta carotene and lycopene are just two of the well known carotenoids without this capability.

There is substantial evidence that most diseases associated with the eyes and brain are the result of oxidation and/or inflammation. Free radicals and singlet oxygen wreak havoc in your head over time, and the consequences, if left unchecked, manifest in such horrible diseases as blindness caused by macular degeneration or dementia caused by Alzheimer's. It is essential that people take antioxidants that can cross the blood-brain and blood-retinal barriers as they get older to protect these vital organs. And it's not just macular degeneration and Alzheimer's to be concerned with, but a whole list of potential problems associated with oxidation and inflammation in the brain and eyes. Below is a list of some of the many detrimental conditions that can develop:

- Glaucoma
- Cataract
- Retinal arterial occlusion
- Venous occlusion
- Diabetic retinopathy
- Age-related macular degeneration

- Injuries resulting from trauma
- Inflammatory injuries
- Alzheimer's disease
- Parkinson's disease
- Huntington's disease
- Amyotrophic lateral sclerosis (Lou Gehrig's disease)
- Senility
- Other forms of age-related dementia

Scientists believe that something may cause people's internal antioxidant defense system to malfunction or wear out as we age. Our bodies may lose the ability to produce high levels of the antioxidants that are normally produced internally such as superoxide dismutase, catalase and glutathione peroxidase. Also, as was pointed out in Chapter 2, our bodies are now subjected to unprecedented levels of oxidation caused by environmental factors such as pollution, contaminants, processed food and the high levels of stress in modern life. All of these lead to an assault on our vital organs as we age, including of course, our brains and eyes.

The eye, in particular, is now subjected to much higher levels of oxidation than our ancestors experienced. The depletion of the ozone layer is causing more intense sunlight than ever before, which directly affects the eyes and skin. Excessive exposure to sunlight and to the highly oxygenated environment causes free radicals to generate in the eye. A condition called "ischemia" which is a type of blockage that deprives the eye of nutrition and oxygen is a common cause of increased oxidation in the eye. Another cause of increased oxidation in the eye happens when the ischemic blockages are removed. The reoxygenation of the tissue after blockage is called "reperfusion," and the end result is another attack on the eye's normal oxidative balance. Even normal enzymatic processes cause increased generation of free radicals and singlet oxygen such as hydrogen peroxide, superoxide and hydroxyl in the eyes.

Free radicals and singlet oxygen oxidize the polyunsaturated fatty acids in the retina which leads to functional impairment of the retinal cell membranes, causing temporary and permanent damage to the retinal cells. Once the retina is damaged, it cannot be replaced. Antioxidants that can reach the inner eye by crossing the blood-brain and blood-retinal barriers are essential because they protect the eye from these damaging conditions.

The carotenoids lutein and zeaxanthin are normally found in the eyes. Astaxanthin is not. We spoke very briefly about groundbreaking work done by

Dr. Mark Tso of the University of Illinois in Chapter 2. Dr. Tso was the first person to prove that Astaxanthin can **cross the blood-brain and blood-retinal barriers**. He took laboratory rats and tested their eyes for Astaxanthin. As expected, he did not find any present. Then he fed the rats Astaxanthin and retested, this time finding Astaxanthin present in the retina. He proved that Astaxanthin could cross first the blood-brain barrier and get into the brain, and then once in the brain it could reach the retina and the macula by crossing through the blood-retinal barrier.

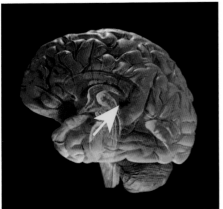

The blood-brain barrier: Astaxanthin can cross through to protect the brain.

Through an extensive series of tests, Dr. Tso went on to prove that Astaxanthin has many protective properties once it reaches the eyes. Among the many benefits that Dr. Tso found include Astaxanthin's ability to protect the eye from:

- Light-induced damage
- Photoreceptor cell damage
- Ganglion cell damage
- Neuronal damage
- Inflammatory damage

Just as with Astaxanthin's anti-inflammatory properties which are a very diverse group of pathways that combat inflammation, the eye-protective properties of Astaxanthin are similar: Astaxanthin protects the eyes through various pathways rather than through just one (Tso, et al, 1996). We see a pattern emerging in which Astaxanthin attacks different problems in a multitude of ways. Perhaps someday researchers will discover that, similar to the case with single pathway anti-inflammatories like Vioxx which have dangerous side effects, this multiple pathway "shotgun" approach to eye health is also the safest and most natural.

Since Dr. Tso's groundbreaking work, other scientists have found further benefits for the eyes when using Natural Astaxanthin. For example, **eye fatigue** is a serious problem in many of today's occupations. Working for long periods at visual display terminals reportedly induces various visual problems such as **eye strain, blurring and diplopia** (a disorder of vision in which two images of a single object are seen because of unequal action of the eye muscles – also called

double vision). In a double blind study performed in Japan, after four weeks of supplementation with 5 mg of Astaxanthin per day (extracted from Haematococcus algae meal) the authors reported a 46% reduction in the number of eye strain subjects. They also found higher accommodation amplitude (the adjustment in the lens of the eye that allows it to focus) in subjects who used visual display terminals. The mechanism of action is still not understood, but it's most likely due to Astaxanthin's potent antioxidant properties (Nagaki, et al, 2002). Additional research in the area of eye fatigue has been carried out. In fact, there are now nine different positive human clinical studies that have been published in the area of eye fatigue.

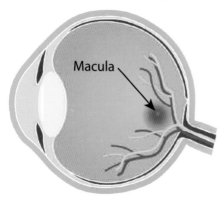

The eye's retina contains the macula. Once damaged, the retina cannot be replaced.

Two different dosage levels were tested for eye fatigue by a group led by Dr. Nakamura in 2004. They found positive effects at 4 mg per day, but found a better result at 12 mg per day (Nakamura, et al, 2004).

Another group of Japanese researchers found similar results in another human clinical study. This double blind study was done to evaluate Astaxanthin's effect on eye fatigue and visual accommodation. Forty subjects were divided into placebo and treatment groups, with the treatment group receiving 6 mg of Astaxanthin for four weeks. The results were that three separate visual parameters were found to have statistically significant benefits from Astaxanthin supplementation. This research established an optimum daily dose for eye fatigue at 6 mg per day (Nitta, et al, 2005).

Additional studies have validated this work, showing that 6 mg per day of Natural Astaxanthin supplementation for four weeks can **reduce eye soreness, dryness, tiredness and blurred vision** (Shiratori, et al, 2005 and Nagaki, et al, 2006).

Astaxanthin may work in a preventive role for eye fatigue as compared to the curative role that has already been established. The other studies referenced above all centered on the use of Astaxanthin to cure eye fatigue. A clinical study was done on subjects whose eyes were healthy, with no signs of fatigue or strain.

40

Both the treatment and the placebo groups were subjected to heavy visual stimuli to induce eye fatigue, and it was found that the treatment group recovered more quickly. This clearly indicates that Natural Astaxanthin may serve to **prevent eye fatigue from occurring in healthy people** (Takahashi and Kajita, 2005).

It is very important to have sufficient blood flow to the eyes and the retina. A human clinical study examined the ability of Astaxanthin to **improve retinal capillary blood flow**. Eighteen subjects were given 6 mg per day of Natural Astaxanthin and another eighteen people were given a placebo. After four weeks it was found that the treatment group had improved retinal capillary blood flow as compared to the placebo group (Yasunori, N, 2005).

The mechanisms of action thought to enable Astaxanthin to reduce or prevent eye fatigue are diverse. Of course, Astaxanthin's role as an antioxidant and anti-inflammatory must play a part. A study conducted at the Hokkaido University Graduate School of Medicine determined that Astaxanthin inhibited inflammation in the eye by blocking nitric oxide synthase (Ohgami, et al, 2003). Astaxanthin was also found to have potent antioxidant effects in the prevention of cataracts in rats' eyes (Wu, et al, 2002). In addition, the increased blood flow to the retina surely plays a part. The final, yet very significant mechanism is improved accommodation amplitude. By enabling the lens to more easily adjust, the ability of the eye to focus is improved.

Another, very different type of human study on Natural Astaxanthin's effects on the eyes has also yielded positive results. This study was done in Japan with subjects comprised of twenty year old men. The treatment group was given 6 mg of Natural Astaxanthin per day for four weeks. Different visual parameters were measured, with statistically significant improvement found in two different parameters for **visual acuity (the ability to see detail)**. The greatest enhancement was seen in **depth perception which improved by 46%** in the group supplementing with Natural Astaxanthin (Sawaki, et al, 2002).

Of course, along with the human clinical trials, there are also pre-clinical animal studies and in-vitro experiments on Astaxanthin and eye health. One such study took the lens from the eyes of pigs and tested the ability of Astaxanthin to protect them from induced oxidative damage. This experiment found that Astaxanthin was capable of **protecting the lens proteins from oxidative damage**. In fact, Astaxanthin performed better than the antioxidant glutathione which is produced by the pig's own body (Wu, et al, 2006).

A study done in rats was very helpful in that it measured the effect of

Astaxanthin on three important inflammatory markers in the uvea (the middle layer of the eye including the iris). Inflammation in the uvea was induced, after which nitric oxide, tumor necrosis factor alpha and prostaglandin E-2 were measured. The rats that had been injected with Astaxanthin had lower levels of all three inflammatory markers. The researchers concluded that Astaxanthin is **effective in reducing ocular inflammation** (Suzuki, et al, 2006). A previous study done on inflammation of the eye of rats yielded similar results, but also demonstrated that the effects of Astaxanthin worked in a dose-dependent fashion. Additionally, this study proved these anti-inflammatory mechanisms in-vitro (Ohgami, et al, 2003).

Less research has been done in direct relation to Astaxanthin's effects on the brain than the extensive work we've cited concerning the eyes, but what has been done is very promising. A series of tests on rodents at the International Research Center for Traditional Medicine in Japan shows great potential. In the first experiment, blood pressure was reduced by the introduction of Astaxanthin to hypertensive rats. Blood pressure is a causative factor for many diseases including some associated with the eyes and brain. The researchers went on to examine the effects of Astaxanthin on stroke prone rats. They found that after five weeks of continuous supplementation, the incidence of stroke was delayed in the treated group. Next, they established a possible mechanism for these results in-vitro, which they believed to be nitric oxide suppression.

The same study went on to demonstrate a **neuroprotective effect (protection of brain function)** in ischemic mice. Ischemia is the condition where there is a deficient supply of blood to the brain as a result of the obstruction of arterial blood flow. In the case of these mice, ischemia was induced by blocking the carotid artery. In humans, this condition can be caused by plaque buildup which can block the flow of blood through the carotid artery in the neck, the primary source of blood to the brain. This build up of plaque can lead to many different maladies including stroke and different types of dementia.

The ischemic mice were fed Astaxanthin only once—just one hour before the ischemia was induced. Remarkable results were seen in the treated group— the mice performed better in a maze designed as a learning performance test. "The present results suggest that Astaxanthin can attenuate the development of hypertension and may help to **protect the brain from stroke and ischemic insults**...In addition, Astaxanthin showed **neuroprotective effects** at relatively high doses by preventing the ischemia-induced impairment of spatial **memory** in mice. This effect is suggested to be due to the significant antioxidant property of

Astaxanthin on ischemia-induced free radicals and their consequent pathological cerebral and neural effects. The current result indicates that Astaxanthin may have beneficial effects in **improving memory in vascular dementia**" (Hussein, et al, 2005a). It appears that Astaxanthin actually **made these mice with restricted blood flow to their brains smarter by improving their memory**. The implications of this study are extremely exciting, as our aging population sees growing numbers of Alzheimer's patients, stroke sufferers and people afflicted by dementia caused by other factors. Further research in humans must be done to fully understand the potential benefit, but these pre-clinical experiments indicate that Astaxanthin may **help sufferers of many brain-related diseases live better lives**.

A similar study had been done previously and was published in Carotenoid Science. This study also demonstrated that Astaxanthin could **prevent brain damage due to ischemia** (Kudo, et al, 2002). A company in Japan did some further work in this area in a rat model. The company fed rats Astaxanthin twice: Twenty four hours before and again one hour before inducing ischemia by occluding the rats' middle arteries. The blood flow stoppage duration was one hour, at which point blood flow to the brain was permitted to resume. The rats were given one more dose of Astaxanthin after blood flow restarted, and then two hours later the rats were sacrificed and their brains were removed. The brains were compared to rats from a control group fed olive oil, and it was found that the **rats fed Astaxanthin had 40% less brain damage** than the control group (Oryza Company, 2006).

Although the research on Astaxanthin's effects on the brain is comprised exclusively of pre-clinical animal studies so far, it is nevertheless very exciting and demonstrates great promise for humans. After seeing the extensive work with Astaxanthin for eye health in human clinical trials, it stands to reason that similar results will be found for brain health as well. This supposition is a logical extension of Astaxanthin's ability to cross the blood-brain and blood-retinal barriers—once in the brain and eyes, Astaxanthin's superior antioxidant properties and anti-inflammatory activity are sure to yield great benefits for these vital organs.

CHAPTER 5

Internal Beauty Pill? Sunscreen in a Pill?

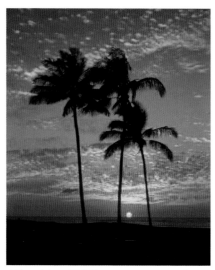

Although beautiful, the sun causes severe damage to unprotected skin

Who would ever think that you can take a pill and it would make you more beautiful from the inside out? Or that this same pill could help protect your skin from UV damage and sunburn? It seems incredible, but there is strong evidence that Natural Astaxanthin can do both. Actually, the two are closely related; the skin is damaged over time by extensive and ongoing exposure to the sun's harmful rays. These ultraviolet rays can cause premature aging of the skin, wrinkles, dry skin, age spots and freckles. By preventing UV damage, skin can be protected from these conditions. And there is evidence that Natural Astaxanthin not only prevents UV damage from occurring, but may actually help to reverse these external signs of aging from the inside out.

Natural Astaxanthin has many great proponents among the medical community. One of them is a doctor and author named Dr. Nicholas Perricone, MD, whose books have appeared on the New York Times best seller list. Dr. Perricone has also appeared on the Oprah Winfrey show twice, and he made sure to talk about Astaxanthin on both occasions. He is a true believer in Natural Astaxanthin—he specifies that people should eat foods that contain the natural variety rather than foods with synthetic Astaxanthin like farm-raised salmon. Perricone's best selling book to date is titled "The Perricone Promise: Look Younger, Live Longer in Three Easy Steps." In this book he devoted three pages to educating his readers about Natural Astaxanthin. In his most recent book, "The

Perricone Weight-Loss Diet," he also extols the virtues of Astaxanthin. He calls it a "Superstar Supplement." He lists a series of benefits for Astaxanthin, two of which are relevant to this chapter: "It provides wrinkle reduction by internal supplementation...It reduces hyperpigmentation (better known as age spots)" (Perricone, N, 2006). On Oprah, Dr. Perricone called Astaxanthin a wonderful anti-inflammatory and antioxidant that "gives you that beautiful, healthy glow."

Dr. Perricone credits Astaxanthin's superior role as an antioxidant to its unique role in protecting the cell membrane. He cites evidence that it has an ability to protect and rejuvenate the skin as an internal beauty supplement. And Dr. Perricone is not the only fan of Astaxanthin from the conventional medical community. Another doctor, although perhaps not as famous as Dr. Perricone, has been raving about Natural Astaxanthin based on his own personal experience.

His name is Dr. Robert Childs, MD. Dr. Childs has been publicly talking about Natural Astaxanthin's many benefits in radio and TV appearances as well as in magazine articles. And it's very interesting to note that he's doing this publicity solely because he's a true believer in Natural Astaxanthin; he receives no compensation from anyone for his appearances. Dr. Childs' personal experience with Natural Astaxanthin is fascinating: Briefly, he was born and raised in Honolulu, Hawaii and was always extremely sensitive to the sun, until he started supplementing with Astaxanthin.

After taking Natural Astaxanthin, Dr. Childs found that he could go out in the midday sun for four hours without burning, as compared to before using Astaxanthin, when he would burn in about a half hour in the intense Hawaiian sun. Dr. Childs says that "BioAstin [a brand of Natural Astaxanthin] literally changed my life, I am outdoors whenever and for as long as I like. For myself, the increased sun tolerance has been quite remarkable." He also found that Astaxanthin helped him with stiffness and soreness in the mornings: "Coincidentally, within a few weeks after I starting taking Astaxanthin, I noticed that it was so much easier to jump out of bed in the morning. The usual stiffness and occasional soreness that would take 15 to 30 minutes to resolve was gone. I didn't think about it much at the time, but looking back at it now, I realize that my physical body regained the smooth, painless functions that I enjoyed in my thirties, almost twenty years ago. Lastly, some of the older surgeons I work with who have confided in me their own "aches and pains" have tried BioAstin themselves and been so amazed that they are now recommending it to their patients." (You can find Dr. Childs' complete testimonial in Chapter 10.)

But even though these two doctors are respected MD's, there still should be clinical proof of Astaxanthin's abilities as an internal beauty supplement and **internal sunscreen**. And there is. In groundbreaking clinical work for which a patent was awarded, Cyanotech Corporation funded a study to test the potential of Natural Astaxanthin as an internal sunscreen. This study was conducted at an independent consumer research laboratory. Twenty one subjects were tested under a solar simulator, a machine designed to emit ultraviolet radiation that mimics sunlight. A filter was used on the machine to ensure ample amounts of both UVA and UVB light reached the subjects' skin.

The skin was tested before supplementation began to see how much UV light was needed to cause erythema (reddening of the skin, a.k.a. sunburn). Then, subjects supplemented with 4 mg of Natural Astaxanthin per day for two weeks. After the two week supplementation period was over, the subjects once again underwent the skin reddening test. The pre-supplementation and post-supplementation scores were then compared. The result was that in only two weeks at a standard dose of just 4 mg per day, there was a statistically significant increase in the amount of time necessary for UV radiation to redden the skin. This result is particularly promising because Astaxanthin has a cumulative effect in the body—it builds up in the organs over time. Two weeks is a relatively short time for the Astaxanthin to concentrate in the body's largest organ, the skin. Yet this study proved that in just two weeks Natural Astaxanthin was already working as an internal sunscreen (Lorenz, T, 2002).

This study did not investigate the mechanism of action for Astaxanthin's abilities as an internal sunscreen, but the answer may not be as complicated as one might think. Sunburn is actually an inflammatory process. When the skin becomes inflamed by exposure to UV light, the inflammation becomes visible through reddening. This is not too different from some other forms of inflammation where the outward appearance manifests as reddening. Swollen ankles, inflamed cuts and abrasions and arthritic hands can all appear red from inflammation. So when our body's largest organ, the skin, turns red, we know that inflammation has taken place. The exact inflammatory pathway or pathways that are being controlled by Astaxanthin's prevention of sunburn are not known; yet it is almost certain that Astaxanthin's anti-inflammatory action is to thank for its action as an internal sunscreen.

There have been animal studies that lend further evidence to Astaxanthin's internal sunscreen indication. Way back in 1995, a study was conducted on special hairless mice to test the protective effects of Astaxanthin, beta carotene or retinol against ultraviolet light. From birth the mice were fed different diets containing combinations of the three substances, the substances alone or a control diet with none of the three substances. After four months, half of each group was exposed to UV light, at which point three markers for skin damage were tested. After irradiation, Astaxanthin alone or in combination with retinol was remarkably effective in **preventing photoaging of the skin** as measured by these markers (Savoure, 1995).

In rat kidney fibroblasts, addition of Astaxanthin demonstrated superior **protection against UVA light-induced oxidative stress** compared to lutein and beta carotene. In fact, Astaxanthin performed at up to 100 times the strength of beta carotene and up to 1000 times the strength of lutein in two different parameters that were measured (O'Connor, I., and O'Brien, N., 1998).

In a study published in the Journal of Dermatological Science, Astaxanthin was tested in-vitro to examine its ability to **protect against alterations in human DNA induced by exposure to UVA radiation**. Three different components of the human skin were tested, and in all three cases Astaxanthin successfully countered the effects of UVA light and prevented damage to the DNA (Lyons, N., and O'Brien, N., 2002).

Astaxanthin can also help **protect the skin from UV damage when applied topically.** A study on hairless mice demonstrated Astaxanthin's topical benefits. The hairless mice were separated into three groups: 1) A control group, 2) a group that would receive UVB radiation after which they would have plain oil that did not contain Astaxanthin put on their skin, and 3) a third group that would receive UVB radiation, after which they would have Astaxanthin in oil put on their skin. The UVB radiation was continued for eighteen weeks to simulate photo aged skin. The results indicated that Astaxanthin reduced wrinkles when compared to the irradiated group that did not have it applied to their skin. And the collagen in the skin in the Astaxanthin treated mice appeared much younger, similar to mice of the same age that had never been exposed to radiation. The study concluded that Astaxanthin can significantly **prevent UV induced collagen degradation and the formation of wrinkles.** "These results suggest that topically applied astaxanthin, which scavenges singlet oxygen effectively, can play an important role to **protect the skin from various photodamages such as lipid peroxidation, sunburn reaction, phototoxicity and photoallergy** induced by singlet oxygen."

The same study examined another benefit from Astaxanthin that is a very marketable one for many countries in Asia. There are a tremendous amount of products known as "skin whiteners" that are sold in several different countries, primarily in East Asia. These products are designed to **reduce melanin**, the substance that can deposit in the skin excessively and cause **freckles, age spots and skin staining**. This study examined Astaxanthin's ability in-vitro to reduce melanin. Astaxanthin was found to decrease melanin production by 40%. This result is superior to three other substances that are commonly included in topical formulas as whitening agents (Arakane, K, 2001).

So we've seen that Astaxanthin can protect hairless mice from UV damage, can decrease melanin production by 40% and can work as an internal sunscreen in humans in just two weeks. Now let's talk about Astaxanthin as an internal beauty supplement. Actually, each of the studies we've already addressed in this chapter lends credibility to Astaxanthin's potential for beauty from within. If Astaxanthin taken internally can prevent UV damage, it will certainly make people's skin look younger and more beautiful. And if it can **decrease melanin production by 40%**, it can help **prevent age spots and freckles.**

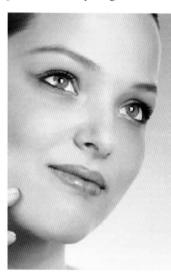

Beauty from within with Natural Astaxanthin

There have now been three studies that have all demonstrated that Natural Astaxanthin taken internally (each time in combination with one or two other nutrients), can have a very positive effect on the way people look. Each combines Astaxanthin with other substances, for example omega 3 fatty acids or a Vitamin E derivative known as tocotrienols, but the common denominator shared by all these studies is that Natural Astaxanthin was present.

The first study in this area was done in Japan. This study combined 2 mg per day of Natural Astaxanthin with tocotrienols (from the Vitamin E family). The study was properly set up as double blind and placebo controlled—neither the subjects nor the researchers knew who was getting a placebo and who was taking the Astaxanthin with tocotrienols. All the subjects were women with an average age of forty. Measurements of several skin parameters were taken after two weeks and again at the end of the study after four weeks. The results were amazing—after just two weeks, improvements were noted in seven different areas:

- Fine wrinkles
- Moisture levels
- Skin tone
- Elasticity
- Smoothness
- Swelling
- Spots and freckles

At such a low level of consumption and in just two weeks, almost every aspect of the treated group's skin was improving! At the end of four weeks, subjects whose skin was characterized as dry at the beginning of the study experienced significantly **increased moisture levels, consistent natural oils, a reduction of fine wrinkles and a reduction of pimples.** On a self-assessment survey, treated subjects reported **less swelling under the eyes, improved elasticity and "better skin feeling."** The placebo group showed no improvements over the four week test period, and in general actually worsened (Yamashita, E., 2002).

The second study was done in Canada, and combined Natural Astaxanthin with two other nutraceuticals, Omega-3 fatty acids and marine glycosaminoglycans. In this study, there were three groups of subjects: The first (Group A) received the active supplement with Astaxanthin, Omega-3's and glycosaminoglycans, and also applied glycosaminoglycans to the skin. The second (Group B) took only the supplement and applied a placebo cream. The third (Group C) applied the glycosaminoglycan cream, but did not take anything orally. The ages of the subjects ranged from 35 – 55, all female, and there were approximately thirty subjects in each group. The study lasted for twelve weeks.

Unfortunately, this study did not measure every parameter for each group. All parameters including **1) fine lines, 2) skin tone, 3) sallowness, 4) roughness, 5) skin elasticity and 6) skin hydration** were measured for Group A, the subjects that used both the supplement and the active cream. Each and every one of these six parameters improved in this group. Additionally, Group A (alone) answered a seventeen point self assessment survey about various aspects of their skin's health before and after the 12 week trial. The regimen met the expectations of 86% of Group A, with general agreement that the regimen was effective in all parameters.

Groups B and C were only tested for two parameters each: Skin elasticity and skin hydration. It was found that Group B (supplement only) had a much better result in skin hydration, while Group C (topical only) had a much better result in skin elasticity. The authors concluded that "Working from the 'inside out' represents a new and exciting cosmeceutical approach to supply the skin with biologically active ingredients" (Thibodeau and Lauzier, 2003). A different study design would have been much more useful for our purposes, but in any event this study is further indication that Natural Astaxanthin may serve as an internal beauty supplement, especially when viewed in relation to the Japanese study previously discussed.

A third study was done in Europe that was very similar to the Japanese study. This one focused exclusively on an internal supplement, this time containing 5 mg per day of Natural Astaxanthin along with two other ingredients. The results were very favorable, with the supplemented group seeing **improvements in fine lines, a visible improvement in overall skin appearance, and an increase in dermis density of up to 78%** in the treatment group. (This study was done on a proprietary formula, and while the authors of this book have been provided with a copy of the study, we have been asked not to disclose the formula or publish the exact details of the study.)

To summarize, Astaxanthin is an effective internal sunscreen that protects the skin from the damage caused by exposure to UV light. This has been demonstrated in-vitro, in animal models as well as in a human clinical trial. In addition to its protective properties, there is evidence that Astaxanthin may have curative properties for the skin and may serve as an internal beauty supplement. More research is necessary in this area. Meanwhile, it certainly appears that Astaxanthin has great potential as an anti-aging supplement.

CHAPTER 6

The Athlete's Secret Weapon

Q. Which of the following can Natural Astaxanthin do for athletes?

A. Make them stronger

B. Give them better stamina

C. Enable them to recover faster

D. Prevent joint and muscle soreness after exercise

E. Plain and simple, make them better athletes

The answer to this question is "all of the above." There is plenty of anecdotal evidence as well as several studies in these areas. Astaxanthin can make you a better athlete. But it's not only for serious athletes; it can also help you during a long Saturday of yard work, or if you're doing aerobics or any other strenuous physical activity. You don't have to be a triathlete like the two gentlemen we mentioned in the first chapter—no matter who you are, if you do any physical activity, hard work or sports, Natural Astaxanthin can help you to do it better and more easily.

Let's take a look at what some athletes say about Natural Astaxanthin:

- Former Competitive Swimmer, Nicholle Davis: "I began taking BioAstin [a brand of Natural Astaxanthin] in May 2002, age 29. I started with one, then two BioAstin daily. It took about four months for my tendonitis to heal to the point that I did not have pain or notice that it was ever there. Now it is November 2004, I'm still taking two BioAstin daily, and still no pain in my shoulders or knees. I have not altered any of my daily routines, diet, or exercise. I directly attribute my use of BioAstin to the healing of

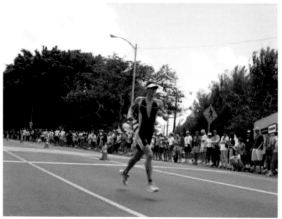

Professional Triathlete Tim Marr, winner of the 2006 Pan American Games Long Distance Triathlon, swears by Natural Astaxanthin.

my tendonitis. I had this condition for 15 years, and nothing I did, didn't do, or tried ever worked.

- Professional Triathlete Tim Marr: "Once I started using BioAstin, I noticed a significant improvement in overuse injuries as well as long term sun exposure. Antioxidants are the secret to training performance and recovery and BioAstin is packed full of high quality antioxidants."

- Former College Wrestler, Mark Vieceli: "I was a collegiate athlete and have had a lot of problems with joint pain in my hands for years. In fact, it gets so bad that I'm unable to hold a newspaper for longer then 5 minutes without my hands and fingers getting sore. I started taking BioAstin about 5 years ago and since taking BioAstin my hands and fingers are 90% better. I started seeing results after the first 2 months. I have tried several different competitive products and within 2 weeks my hands were just as bad as prior to taking BioAstin. I will definitely never use anything else! I'm glad I finally found something that works."

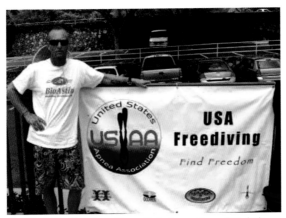

America's Top Freediver, Deron Verbeck, sporting a "BioAstin Natural Astaxanthin" T-shirt

- America's Top Freediver, Deron Verbeck: "Once I started taking BioAstin I noticed an overall change in my health. I was getting sick far less than previous years. Colds and flu, which are a potential problem for freediving during training and for competition as I push my body to its limits, had become a non-issue for me. On top of this I was noticing changes in my training itself. During dives I found that on my ascent I was getting far less fatigued and absolutely no lactic acid build up in my quadriceps. I was also recovering from the dives much quicker on the surface, which means that I am able to catch my breath far quicker than before."

- Marathon Runner, Dien Truong: "Taking the BioAstin made a huge difference in my recovery time as well as allowing me to run pain free on my daily training runs of 6 miles."

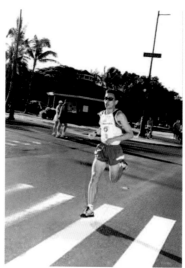

Hawaii's Top Marathon Runner and avid
fan of Natural Astaxanthin, Jonathan Lyau

- Hawaii's Top Marathon Runner, Jonathan Lyau: "Marathon training is very demanding and BioAstin has helped me recover from intense workouts quicker even though I was getting older. I also found that I no longer needed to take various antioxidants or glucosamine as BioAstin seemed to have benefits of these supplements too."

(**Note:** The above are excerpts from what athletes wrote about their experience with Natural Astaxanthin. Their full testimonials are available in Chapter 10.)

Many athletes feel very strongly about Natural Astaxanthin, but as you can see, it's for a variety of different reasons. In the Anti-Inflammatory chapter we looked at several studies that all showed how Natural Astaxanthin can help reduce aches and pains triggered by inflammation. As we noted, inflammation is a normal process in the body which can be caused by many different things. But inflammation can slow an athlete down, and can prevent athletes from recovering quickly, which is very undesirable, as this prevents them from having frequent workouts. The athletes quoted above talk about faster recovery, less pain and reduction in overuse injuries. They also say that Astaxanthin helps them with tendonitis and long term joint pain. And one of the world's top freedivers is experiencing less fatigue during dives because of Astaxanthin. If you take the time to read through all the many testimonials from around the world in Chapter 10, you'll see people from all walks of life that swear that Natural Astaxanthin has helped them to work much harder and longer, to have pain free workouts and fast recoveries, to become stronger—pretty much all the things that the salmon swimming upstream for a week straight is experiencing. Natural Astaxanthin is truly the "Athlete's Secret Weapon." Now, let's study the science that shows how and why this is so.

Briefly, we should start by taking a quick refresher on what we've already learned about how Natural Astaxanthin can help athletes, based on studies that we've already discussed. We've seen that Natural Astaxanthin:

- Improves grip strength in sufferers of tennis elbow (tendonitis) by 93% in just eight weeks
- Eliminates joint soreness after exercise
- Assists in the reduction of pain from various inflammatory causes
- Works as an internal sunscreen and protects the skin from UV light (especially important for athletes training outdoors)

One of the most important benefits that Natural Astaxanthin has for athletes or people working or playing hard is that it actually increases strength and endurance. Remember the salmon? It appears that this same effect of Astaxanthin concentrating in the muscles occurs in humans. A very exciting study in Sweden back in 1998 verified what early users of Natural Astaxanthin were reporting—that they were getting stronger and increasing their endurance when supplementing with Astaxanthin. The study was done with healthy male students between the ages of seventeen and nineteen. The researcher used forty men with an equal number (twenty) in the treatment group and in the placebo group. Each subject took one 4 mg capsule per day with a meal for six months.

The subjects' strength was measured at the beginning of the experiment, halfway through (after three months), and again at the end of the experiment (after six months). The strength test was scientifically designed: They measured the maximum number of knee bends to a 90° angle that each subject could do. This was controlled by an adjustable stool in a "Smith machine." (The Smith machine is specifically designed for measuring strength and endurance in clinical trials.) The subjects were properly warmed up for a set time and in a similar manner before each strength measurement.

The results were truly amazing: In six months, the students taking Natural Astaxanthin improved **their strength and endurance by 62%**! And this at the relatively low dose of only 4 mg per day. The students taking a placebo increased their strength by 22%, which is normal for people in this age group over a six

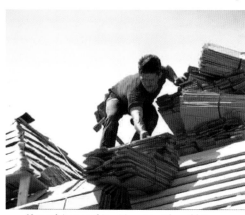

month period, as they were generally involved in sports and physically activity. So basically, Astaxanthin made these students stronger and **increased their endurance three times faster** than the placebo group! (Malmsten, 1998). While these same results cannot be guaranteed for older people or even for people in the same age groups, they certainly indicate that Astaxanthin increases strength and endurance. It makes sense that any athlete who under-

Natural Astaxanthin—it's not just for athletes

stands that Natural Astaxanthin is completely safe and hears these results would want to try it for themselves. In fact, even without all the other benefits for athletes, the competitive edge that Natural Astaxanthin can give for strength and endurance is a huge advantage in and of itself.

Let's look at how Astaxanthin helps in this area: Mitochondrial cells, many of which are found in muscle tissue, produce up to 95% of our body's energy by burning fatty acids and other substances. But this energy that is produced also generates highly reactive free radicals. The free radicals, in turn, damage cell membranes and oxidize DNA. And the free radicals continue to impact the muscles even after we stop exercising—they activate inflammatory markers which lodge in muscle tissue and cause soreness and tiredness.

According to the mitochondrial theory of aging, degradation done to the mitochondria is due largely to oxidative damage. The damage done in the cells leaves the mitochondria deficient of respiration and inefficient in producing energy. When a cell is no longer producing energy optimally, the strength and endurance of the individual declines.

Because Astaxanthin is such a powerful antioxidant, it effectively **scavenges the muscle tissue for free radicals and eliminates singlet oxygen.**

During all strenuous physical activity, the body produces large amounts of free radicals. The more strenuous the activity, the greater the production of free radicals. (For example, when the body is consuming oxygen at 70% above the average rate, a rate that is quite common in endurance exercise and aerobics, there are approximately twelve times the amount of free radicals in the cells as when the person is resting.) It is probable that the mechanism of action that enables Natural Astaxanthin to make people stronger and increase their endurance is through its intense **antioxidant and anti-inflammatory activity in the energy-producing mitochondria.**

A different kind of sports-related clinical study was done in Japan to measure Natural Astaxanthin's effect on lactic acid levels in the muscles. Lactic acid is an unwanted byproduct of physical exertion; it deposits in the muscles and causes burning during exercise. The **result of reducing lactic acid levels is increased endurance.**

This study was also done with young men, all twenty years old; the treatment group took 6 mg per day of Natural Astaxanthin for four weeks. Lactic acid levels for both groups were measured before running 1200 meters and again two minutes after running. The results were very positive: The young men taking

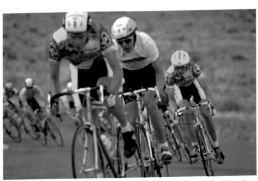

Heavy exercise generates up to 12X the normal levels of free radicals

Natural Astaxanthin **averaged 28.6% lower serum lactic acid** after running 1200 meters compared to the placebo group (Sawaki, et al, 2002).

A fascinating health survey was completed in 2001 which investigated the effects of Astaxanthin on exercise. The survey involved 247 people between 20 and 87 years of age. Out of these, 146 reported problems with muscle and joint soreness. After compiling the data, an amazing pattern was discovered: When taking Astaxanthin, **88% of all participants reported improvement in muscle and joint soreness.** In all cases, the more exercise an individual did, the more benefit was experienced (Guerin, et al, 2002).

In addition to these two positive human clinical trials and this encouraging exercise survey, two additional clinical trials that we've already mentioned have a direct relevance for athletes. In the study we discussed in Chapter 4 relating to Natural Astaxanthin's ability to **improve visual acuity**, it is important to note that this trial was done on handball enthusiasts before and after a handball workout. Astaxanthin helped them with visual acuity in two different areas, with the greatest benefit in **depth perception (an improvement of 46%)**. In handball as well as in many other sports, depth perception is vital to success (Sawaki, et al, 2002).

The second study that we talked about earlier that has direct relevance for athletes was the joint soreness clinical at the University of Memphis. The researcher for this study, Dr. Fry, reexamined the data well after the original paper was submitted and found an interesting, novel result: A certain subset of the men in this trial that were training with weights found **reduced muscle soreness** as well as the absence of joint soreness that was originally reported (Fry, et al, 2004). In addition to Dr. Fry's findings, Astaxanthin's potential to reduce muscle soreness after exercise is backed up by a great deal of anecdotal evidence, but this benefit should be studied in more depth in additional trials with larger and more diverse subject pools.

Of course, there are animal studies that corroborate the human clinical proof cited above. One such study done with mice was designed to measure the effects of Astaxanthin on endurance. The results were similar to the endurance clinical in young men: **Astaxanthin markedly increased endurance** in mice.

This study took course over a five week period. Mice were divided into two groups and their endurance was tested by seeing how long they could swim until exhaustion. The mice fed Astaxanthin showed a **significant increase in swimming time before exhaustion** than the control group. **Blood lactose levels** were measured in both groups, and, as expected, the levels of the Astaxanthin group were significantly lower than the control group. Another effect measured was fascinating: Astaxanthin supplementation **significantly reduced fat accumulation**. This is the first mention of such an effect and further proof is needed before putting any credence into this potential benefit. The study's authors suggested that Astaxanthin enabled the mitochondria to burn more fat: "These results suggest that improvement in swimming endurance by the administration of astaxanthin is caused by an increase in utilization of fatty acids as an energy source" (Ikeuchi, et al, 2006). It's very interesting to note that the results of this mouse study exactly reiterate the human clinical trials—**Astaxanthin increases endurance and reduces lactic acid levels**.

The last study we'll examine in this chapter was completed in Japan at the

Kyoto University of Medicine. This study took mice and ran them on a treadmill until they were exhausted. The mice were separated into three different groups: Group A was the control group that was not exercised at all and was not given Astaxanthin. Group B was exercised until exhaustion, but was not given Astaxanthin either. Group C was exercised similarly to Group B, but their diets were supplemented with Natural Astaxanthin. After the exhaustive exercise, the mice were sacrificed and examined. Their heart muscles and calf muscles were checked for oxidative damage. The researchers found that various **markers of oxidative damage were reduced in both the heart muscles and calf muscles** of Group C. They found a corresponding **reduction of oxidation in the plasma** as well. The **cell membranes** in the treatment group's calf and heart muscles suffered significantly **less peroxidation damage**. Also, **damage to DNA and proteins were significantly reduced** in the mice supplemented with Astaxanthin. Another effect noticed was **better modulation of inflammation damage indicators and serum creatine kinase**. In fact, **muscle inflammation was found to decrease by more than 50%** in the mice given Astaxanthin. "Our data documented that astaxanthin indeed is absorbed and transported into skeletal muscle and heart in mice, even though most carotenoids accumulate mainly in the liver and show relatively little distribution to other peripheral tissues, including skeletal muscle and heart. This unique pharmacokinetic characteristic of astaxanthin makes it well suited to oxidative stress in gastrocnemius [calf] and heart…Thus, astaxanthin attenuates exercise-induced damage by directly scavenging reactive oxygen species and also by down-regulating the inflammatory response" (Aoi, et al, 2003).

This study proves, first of all, by examining the calf muscles and heart muscles of mice, that Natural Astaxanthin actually reaches these two very spread out areas in the rodents' bodies. The authors point out that this is not the case with most other carotenoids. This is a unique and very important difference between Natural Astaxanthin and other antioxidants and carotenoids: Many cannot get throughout the body. Because of its shape and esterified nature (with fatty acids attached to one or both ends of the molecule), Natural Astaxanthin has this tremendous advantage—it **travels to the far reaches of the body, into every organ**—the brain, the heart, the muscles and even the skin, fighting oxidation and inflammation and thereby protecting them.

The other key point that this study proved was that, once in these diverse areas of the body, Astaxanthin was doing exactly what it's supposed to do—**eliminating free radicals, reducing inflammation and preventing damage to DNA**

and cell membranes. This is one of the most significant animal studies to date demonstrating the extensive and varied benefits of Natural Astaxanthin in-vivo.

In conclusion, it's easy to see that the combination of benefits such as 1) strength and endurance building, 2) joint and muscle soreness prevention after exercise, 3) faster recovery, 4) anti-inflammatory and antioxidant protection of the energy-producing mitochondria and 5) reduced damage to the cell membranes and DNA would make Natural Astaxanthin a powerful weapon in any athlete's arsenal.

CHAPTER 7

Other Medical Research

Natural Astaxanthin is a powerful antioxidant and a safe, natural anti-inflammatory. It protects the skin from UV damage and helps make people more beautiful from the inside out. It's a great supplement for athletes and active people, helping with recovery from exercise, helping to prevent joint soreness after exercise and even making people stronger and giving them increased endurance. It's a wonderful aid to the eyes and brain, and helps prevent such diseases as macular degeneration and cataracts.

But Natural Astaxanthin doesn't just help in these areas. In fact, there are indications from some human clinical trials as well as strong evidence from animal studies that Natural Astaxanthin may help in several other ways.

Immune System Support

There has been some promising research on the effects of Natural Astaxanthin in enhancing immunity. A series of studies were conducted during the 1990's by Dr. Jyonouchi and various associates, first at the University of South Florida and later at the University of Minnesota's School of Medicine. The first study was in-vitro work on mouse and sheep blood, in which Astaxanthin was shown to have an immunomodulating effect as compared to beta carotene (which did not). "These results indicate that immunomodulating actions of carotenoids are not necessarily related to pro-vitamin A activity, because astaxanthin, which does not have pro-vitamin A activity, showed more significant effects" (Jyonouchi, et al, 1991). A follow up study in 1993 examined the mechanism of action for Astaxanthin's immunomodulating effects, and found it is related to enhancement of antibody production to T-cell dependent antigen (Jyonouchi, et al, 1993).

The following year, Dr. Jyonouchi went one step further by examining these in-vitro effects in live mice, and compared the effects of Astaxanthin this time with both beta carotene and lutein. The outcome was that all three carotenoids had significant immunomodulating action. In a group of old mice, Astaxanthin stood out beyond its carotenoid cousins as it partially restored antibody production to a greater extent than did lutein and beta carotene (Jyonouchi, et al, 1994).

The next study in this series was done in-vitro using samples from the blood of adult (human) volunteers, as well as blood from the umbilical cord of newborn babies. Testing was done with both beta carotene and Astaxanthin to check if they could increase immune markers in the blood. It was found that beta carotene had no effect, while Astaxanthin increased the production of two different forms of immunoglobulin. The researchers concluded: "This study has shown for the first time that astaxanthin, a carotenoid without vitamin A activity, enhances human immunoglobulin production in response to T-dependent stimuli" (Jyonouchi, et al, 1995).

The final study in this series measured Astaxanthin's and several other carotenoids' potency as immune enhancers. Astaxanthin did considerably more at equal dosage levels than all other carotenoids, including lutein, lycopene, zeaxanthin and canthaxanthin. Astaxanthin alone suppressed interferon-gamma production and increased the number of antibody-secreting cells with the use of primed spleen cells. In another test, only Astaxanthin and zeaxanthin had a positive result (Jyonouchi, et al, 1996).

Similar work was done the same year in Japan by other researchers, where Astaxanthin was again tested against beta carotene and canthaxanthin. Once again, it was found that Astaxanthin enhanced two different forms of immunoglobulin; canthaxanthin had a moderate effect and beta carotene had a slight effect at much higher doses. The release of inflammatory markers TNF-a and IL-1a was also enhanced. The summary ranked the cytokine inducing activities in this order: Astaxanthin>canthaxanthin>beta carotene. "These results indicate that carotenoids such as beta carotene, canthaxanthin and astaxanthin have possible immunomodulating activities to enhance the proliferation and functions of murine immunocompetent cells" (Okai and Higashi-Okai, 1996).

Another slant on the immune benefits of Astaxanthin is seen in a study involving Helicobacter pylori, a bacterium commonly found in the stomach that can lead to cancer. There is quite a bit of data on Astaxanthin's effects on H. pylori, which we'll examine later in this chapter. In this particular study, the author states that "Recent experimental studies, both in vivo and in vitro, have shown that vitamin C and astaxanthin, a carotenoid, are not only free radical scavengers but also show antimicrobial activity against H. pylori. It has been shown that astaxanthin changes the immune response to H. pylori by shifting the Th1 response towards a Th2 T-cell response" (Akyon, Y, 2002). Because Astaxanthin can actually change the immune response, it is very effective at reducing H. pylori, which can help prevent certain types of gastric cancer and other stomach ailments.

B.P. Chew, PhD, a professor at Washington State University, has also been studying Astaxanthin's effects on the immune system. First he looked at how Astaxanthin boosted immunity in mice. He discovered that Astaxanthin and beta carotene both increased the lymphocyte function in mice's spleens. This was not true of canthaxanthin. Astaxanthin had an additional positive effect that beta carotene did not in that it also enhanced lymphocyte cytotoxic activity.

After proving immune system enhancement in mice, Dr. Chew moved on to study the effect in humans. In a double blind, placebo controlled human clinical, Dr. Chew and his team showed that Astaxanthin is a strong immune system stimulator. The study showed that Astaxanthin:

- Stimulates lymphocyte proliferation
- Increases the total number of antibody producing B-cells
- Produces increased number of T-cells
- Amplifies natural killer cell cytotoxic activity
- Significantly increases delayed-type hypersensitivity response
- Dramatically decreases DNA damage

For those who are not scientists, this basically shows that Astaxanthin works in many different ways to support healthy immune function in humans (Chew, et al, 2003). It appears that, similar to the various pathways that Astaxanthin uses to attack inflammation, it also uses various pathways to boost immunity.

Dr. Chew, along with Dr. J.S. Park, wrote a summary article entitled "Carotenoid Action on the Immune Response" in which they spoke very highly of Astaxanthin's advantages for tumor immunity. They stated that "Even though astaxanthin, canthaxanthin and beta carotene inhibited tumor growth, astaxanthin showed the highest anti-tumor activity" (Chew and Park, 2004). We'll study Astaxanthin's role as a cancer preventive and treatment in more detail later in this chapter.

Cardiovascular Benefits

Natural Astaxanthin is a very good tonic for the heart. It has a variety of properties that can **help people prevent heart disease** and also help people with heart disease to **minimize their risk of a heart attack or stroke**. The antioxidant power and the ability to reduce silent inflammation are two obvious cardiovascular benefits that were addressed in earlier chapters, but there are a few additional potential benefits that have been demonstrated in human clinical trials and/or pre-clinical animal studies.

There is evidence that Natural Astaxanthin can help **improve blood lipid profiles by decreasing low density lipoprotein (LDL, bad cholesterol) and triglycerides, and by increasing high density lipoprotein (HDL, good cholesterol).** This has been demonstrated in both human and animal trials.

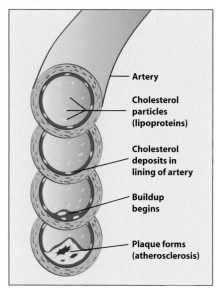

Artery

Cholesterol particles (lipoproteins)

Cholesterol deposits in lining of artery

Buildup begins

Plaque forms (atherosclerosis)

*From healthy arteries to clogged arteries—
the formation of plaque*

An early study in rats demonstrated that Astaxanthin **raised HDL**, the good cholesterol (Murillo, E, 1992). A later study tested both Astaxanthin and Vitamin E in rabbits that had high cholesterol. This research found that both supplements, particularly Astaxanthin, **improved plaque stability in the arteries**. All the rabbits that ingested Astaxanthin were classified as "early plaques," as compared to the rabbits ingesting Vitamin E and also the control group (Li, et al, 2004). A third animal study was done recently in rats. This study showed that Astaxanthin increased HDL while decreasing both triglycerides and non-esterified fatty acids in the blood (Hussein, et al, 2006).

A human clinical trial in Japan found a very **promising effect on LDL** (bad cholesterol) both in test tubes and in human volunteers. The in-vitro test showed that Astaxanthin dose-dependently prolonged the oxidation lag time of LDL. The test was then repeated in humans at doses as low as 1.8 mg per day and as high as 21.6 mg per day for fourteen days. This study found that all four doses positively affected LDL oxidation lag time—at 1.8 mg per day it was 5% longer; at 3.6 mg it was 26% longer; at 14.4 mg it was 42% longer; and at the highest dose of 21.6 mg, the upward trend stopped and the lag time was only 31% longer. This suggests that the optimum dose for blood lipid profiles is significantly less than 21.6 mg per day. The researchers concluded that consumption of Astaxanthin "inhibits LDL oxidation and possibly therefore contributes to the **prevention of atherosclerosis**" (Iwamoto, et al, 2000).

An unpublished human clinical trial was done in Eastern Europe on men with high cholesterol. Subjects supplemented with 4 mg of Astaxanthin (as BioAstin®) for thirty days. At the end of the study, subjects taking Astaxanthin showed an average **decrease in total cholesterol and of LDL of 17%, and an average decrease of triglycerides of 24%!** (Trimeks, 2003).

Another potential benefit for cardiovascular health may be Astaxanthin's ability to **decrease blood pressure**. To date, research has been only pre-clinical animal trials in rodents, but the results look promising. A group of Japanese researchers have done three separate experiments on rats with high blood pressure. In the first study, the researchers discovered that supplementation with Astaxanthin for fourteen days resulted in a significant decrease in blood pressure for the hypertensive rats, while rats with normal blood pressure levels showed no decrease. They also showed that stroke-prone rats that were fed Astaxanthin for five weeks had a **delayed incidence of stroke** while also decreasing their blood pressure. This research was part of the study referenced in the "Eyes and Brain" chapter, where mice with poor blood flow to the brain proved to be smarter after being fed Astaxanthin. The study concluded, "These results indicate that astaxanthin can exert beneficial effects in **protection against hypertension and stroke and in improving memory in vascular dementia**." This study was very broad in its scope and quite ground-breaking (Hussein, et al, 2005a), so the same researcher led another study later the same year.

The second study again examined the effect of Astaxanthin on hypertensive rats, but with an aim of also finding **Astaxanthin's mechanism of action for high blood pressure**. They found that Astaxanthin's mechanism for decreasing high blood pressure may be its modulating effect on nitric oxide. As discussed in Chapter 3, nitric oxide is also a causative factor for inflammation. So at the same time Astaxanthin is controlling inflammation through its modulation of nitric oxide, it is also controlling blood pressure. This study went on to examine the hearts of the rats after contractions were induced with a variety of substances.

The constrictive effects of these introduced substances were improved by Astaxanthin, demonstrating that it may help **reduce the consequences of a heart attack**. The conclusion was that Astaxanthin may **help with blood fluidity** in hypertension, and that it may **restore the vascular tone** (Hussein, et al, 2005b).

With two groundbreaking studies under his belt, Dr. Hussein led his team at the Institute of Natural Medicine in Japan to another outstanding study in 2006. This study was already cited above, in reference to cholesterol, as the rats that were fed Astaxanthin increased their HDL and decreased their triglycerides and non-esterified fatty acids. Again, the subject rats were hypertensive, and again, results showed that Astaxanthin reduced blood pressure in hypertensive rats. A very interesting sideline of this study was a positive effect on key indicators of diabetes as well, which we'll examine later in this chapter (Hussein, et al, 2006). All of us in the study of Natural Astaxanthin sincerely hope that Dr. Hussein will continue his exceptional work.

There is one human study that is related to this anti-hypertensive animal research as well as the blood lipid research. This study centered on human volunteers supplementing with 6 mg of Astaxanthin per day for only ten days. At the end of the ten day period, a **significant improvement in blood flow** was found in the treatment group (Miyawaki, H, 2005).

A very different type of animal study related to cardiac health was done by a different group of Japanese scientists at the Kyoto University of Medicine. We talked about this study in Chapter 6. The study found that mice that were fed Astaxanthin and then run on a treadmill until exhaustion suffered **less heart damage** than mice that were similarly exercised without Astaxanthin supplementation. On examination, they found Astaxanthin concentrated in the mice's hearts. They concluded that Astaxanthin can **decrease exercise induced damage in the heart** as well as in the skeletal muscle (Aoi, et al, 2003).

At the Medical College of Wisconsin, another animal study with rats showed cardio-protective attributes for Astaxanthin. In this study, Astaxanthin was given to rats prior to heart attacks. It was found that Astaxanthin significantly **reduced the area of infarction and the damage caused to the heart by the heart attack** (Gross and Lockwood, 2004).

Lastly, let's briefly talk about a group of researchers from Honolulu, Hawaii that are looking at making a unique, injectable delivery system for Astaxanthin into a patented prescription drug for cardiovascular patients. The group has trademarked the name Cardax® for their product and has done extensive research on it. Three of these studies are of particular interest: In the first, they used rats as the model for their experiment and in the second they used dogs. Both results were very promising: "These results suggest that Cardax has marked **cardioprotective properties** in both rodents and canines. Thus, Cardax may be a novel and powerful new means to **prevent myocardial [inner heart muscle tissue] injury**" (Gross and Lockwood, 2003 and 2005).

The third study that was done on Cardax was extremely exciting. It was led by a scientist at the prestigious Harvard Medical School. This study tested Cardax's effect on the negative side effects of Vioxx®. As we mentioned in the first chapter, Vioxx is a prescription anti-inflammatory that can have a horrible

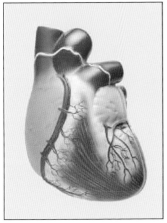

The human heart—protected many different ways by Astaxanthin

side effect of causing deaths from cardiovascular disease and heart attacks. This study states that the dangerous cardiovascular effects that may be caused by Vioxx are related to its action of increasing the susceptibility of LDL and cellular membrane lipids to oxidation, which contributes to plaque instability and thrombus formation (formation of blood clots in the arteries). This study demonstrated that Vioxx is a pro-oxidant. Now for the amazing part: Astaxanthin, as an antioxidant, **completely negated the pro-oxidant effect of Vioxx**! The study states, "Remarkably, astaxanthin was able to completely inhibit the adverse effects of Vioxx on lipid peroxidation…We have now demonstrated a pharmacologic approach to block the pro-oxidant effects of Vioxx using a high lipophilic chain-breaking antioxidant, astaxanthin" (Mason, et al, 2006).

The work that is being done on Cardax, the unique injectable delivery system for Astaxanthin, shows tremendous potential, but you don't have to wait for this to become an approved, prescription drug. The medical research to date clearly demonstrates that Natural Astaxanthin, already available as a low cost dietary supplement in most countries, has many diverse cardiovascular benefits as well.

Ulcers, Gastric Injury, Stomach Cancer

There's a very destructive bacteria found in about half of the world population's stomach called Helicobacter pylori. H. pylori's initial manifestation is in the form of chronic gastritis and stomach ulcers. Left untreated it can lead to more serious consequences including stomach cancer and lymphoma. It can be caused by eating a diet deficient in some very important nutrients such as carotenoids. "A low dietary intake of antioxidants such as carotenoids and Vitamin C may be an important factor for the acquisition of H. pylori by humans" (Bennedsen, et al, 1999). One study was cited previously in this chapter in which Astaxanthin was shown to be able to change the immune response to H. pylori (Akyon, Y, 2002). Other studies have demonstrated that Astaxanthin has a positive effect on H. Pylori and the gastrointestinal system. Two studies were done in Scandinavia using Natural Astaxanthin on H. pylori-infected mice. The first, in Denmark, found that an Astaxanthin-rich algae extract reduced the bacterial load and gastric inflammation (Bennedsen, et al, 1999). The second study which was done in Sweden, showed results both in test tubes and in live mice. Natural Astaxanthin in algae meal inhibited the growth of H. pylori in-vitro. In the ex-vivo part of this study, the mice that ate the Haematococcus algae meal showed lower bacteria levels and lower inflammation scores than untreated or control-meal treated mice when tested one day after as well as ten days after the cessation of treatment (Wang, et al, 2000).

Two studies done at Korea University by researcher J.H. Kim, PhD and associates tested Astaxanthin's ability to prevent the gastric damage caused by 1) naproxen and 2) ethyl alcohol. In the first study, the non-steroidal anti-inflammatory drug naproxen was given to rats. Naproxen is known to cause ulcerative lesions in the stomach. Rats fed Astaxanthin at three different dosage levels all realized significant protection against naproxen's deleterious effects on the stomach lining. Also noted was that pretreatment with Astaxanthin significantly increased the activities of free radical scavenging enzymes super oxide dismutase (SOD), catalase and glutathione peroxidase. "These results suggest that astaxanthin removes the lipid peroxides and free radicals induced by naproxen, and it may offer potential remedy of gastric ulceration" (Kim, et al, 2005a). Dr. Kim's second study involved ethyl alcohol, the active ingredient in whiskey, rum, vodka, etc. that can cause ulcerative gastric lesions in humans when consumed in excess. Once again, rats were used, and once again, similar results were found. As with Astaxanthin's effects on naproxen, its effects on ethyl alcohol showed significant protection against ulcers, and pretreatment increased the free radical scavenging activities of SOD, catalase and glutathione peroxidase. "A histologic examination clearly indicated that the acute gastric mucosal lesion induced by ethanol nearly disappeared after pretreatment with astaxanthin" (Kim, et al, 2005b).

The last study we'll look at in this section was done in Japan, and it is very interesting in that it tested three different forms of Astaxanthin—Natural Astaxanthin from Haematococcus microalgae, Astaxanthin from the mutated yeast Phaffia Rhodiza, and Astaxanthin synthesized from petrochemicals—along with Vitamin C and beta carotene, on their ulcer preventative abilities in stressed rats. Rats were subjected to two different types of stress that cause ulcers. The rats fed all forms of Astaxanthin as well as beta carotene were appreciably protected from the formation of gastric ulcerations. However, an extremely significant result of this research was that "Ulcer indexes in particular were smaller with the rat group fed astaxanthin extracted from Haematococcus than the other groups." The research further showed that by combining Astaxanthin and Vitamin C "protected against the evolution of gastric ulcerations in relation to control rats. The effects were more intense, especially in rats simultaneously supplied Astaxanthin and Vitamin C...the simultaneous supplementation of food substances with Astaxanthin and Vitamin C would supply enough antioxidants to offset stress-related injuries" (Nishikawa, et al, 2005). This study is more vital evidence of the superiority of Natural Astaxanthin to other forms, as well as another piece of science demonstrating efficacy for Astaxanthin in gastrointestinal health.

Detoxification

The liver and kidneys help to detoxify the body by removing harmful substances. One of the key functions of the liver is the active oxidation of fats to produce energy. The liver also can destroy pathogenic bacteria and viruses, and can eliminate dead red blood cells. All of these various functions can initiate the release of high volumes of free radicals. It is very important to have the protective influence of neutralizing antioxidants in the liver to combat this ongoing oxidative process.

One study examined the protective effects of Astaxanthin versus Vitamin E of rat liver cells against lipid peroxidation. It was found that Astaxanthin was a much more effective antioxidant for these liver cells (Kurashige, et al, 1990). Astaxanthin also has the beneficial effect of causing the liver to produce certain enzymes that may help prevent the formation of liver cancer (Gradelet, et al, 1998). And in the kidneys and lungs, Astaxanthin was also shown to have a similar effect of inducing the release of these beneficial enzymes. So, not only can Astaxanthin help the detoxifying organs counter the oxidizing effects of free radicals, but at the same time it can promote the release of beneficial enzymes. Liver benefits were also seen in a rat study in 2001, where Astaxanthin's antioxidant properties appeared to protect the rats from liver damage. A measurable increase in superoxide dismutase (SOD) and glutathione was found in the rats' livers (Kang, et al, 2001).

Cancer Prevention and Tumor Reduction

First, let's start by saying that there is no evidence that Astaxanthin can prevent cancer or reduce tumors in humans. But there sure is plenty of evidence for these benefits in animals. Strictly speaking, we can't imply that Astaxanthin's effects on preventing cancer and reducing tumor sizes in animals such as rodents means that it will have the same effects in humans; these are preclinical trials designed to show if the possibility exists. But it seems logical based on over 200 epidemiological studies on reduced levels of cancers in people whose diets include high levels of natural beta carotene, Natural Astaxanthin's carotenoid cousin (Moorhead, et al, 2006, Zhang, et al, 1999, Holick, et al, 2002, and Rock, C, 2003); if beta carotene helps prevent cancer, and Astaxanthin is 11 – 50 times stronger as an antioxidant than beta carotene, then perhaps Astaxanthin will be much stronger in preventing cancer as well. Indeed, many fruits and vegetables are known to help prevent carcinogenesis, so it isn't too surprising that a natural vegetable supplement like Natural Astaxanthin might have these same properties (Wargovich, M, 1997, Potter, J, 1997 and Eastwood, M, 1999). And because Natural Astaxanthin is a concentrated vegetable extract, it wouldn't be surprising if it worked much better than fruits and vegetables.

Unless you eat a lot of salmon on a regular basis, or a whole lot of crab, lobster or shrimp, you're probably not going to have a measurable amount of Astaxanthin in your blood (unless, of course, you take a Natural Astaxanthin supplement). This makes it much more difficult to test the epidemiological effects of Astaxanthin. One interesting point to note epidemiologically is the unusually low incidence of cancer in certain indigenous populations that eat large amounts of salmon on a regular basis, such as the Eskimos and certain coastal tribes in North America (Bates, et al, 1985).

Let's look at some cancer research with Astaxanthin: The anti-carcino-genic research for Astaxanthin has been limited thus far to in-vitro work and animal studies. In one in-vitro study, mouse tumor cells were put into a solution supplemented with Astaxanthin and into the same solution without Astaxanthin. After one and two days, it was found that the tumor cells in the Astaxanthin solution had lower cell numbers as well as a lower DNA synthesis rate (Sun, et al, 1998). In another study of mouse breast tumor cells, it was found that Astaxanthin reduced the proliferation of the tumor cells by 40% in a dose-dependent fashion (Kim, et al, 2001). A very interesting study pitted Astaxanthin against eight other carotenoids to see which was most effective at inhibiting liver tumor cells in culture. It was found that Astaxanthin surpassed every other carotenoid in this test (Kozuki, 2000).

The proliferation of human cancer cell lines has also been inhibited by Astaxanthin in vitro. Human colon cancer cell lines were placed in a culture containing Astaxanthin versus one that was Astaxanthin free. After four days, the cell lines in the culture containing Astaxanthin were significantly less viable (Onogi, et al, 1998). Also, in work with human prostate cancer cells, Astaxanthin and lycopene both showed significant inhibitory effects (Levy, et al, 2002).

So, we know that Astaxanthin has chemo-preventative effects in test tubes. Now let's look at the effects in small mammals. In one study, researchers transplanted tumor cells into mice and found that Astaxanthin inhibited the growth of the cancerous tumors, again in a dose-dependent fashion (Sun, et al, 1998). A similar study was done to see at what stage the Astaxanthin would have its positive effects. It was found that when Astaxanthin supplementation was started both at one week and also at three weeks prior to the tumor inoculation, growth was inhibited. However, when the supplementation with Astaxanthin began at the same time as the tumor inoculation, the benefit was not found. The conclusion of this study was that Astaxanthin may work better in the early stages of tumor development, but not in the later stages. The researcher was very enthused with Astaxanthin's potential in cancer prevention, pointing out that the anti-tumor activity came at blood concentration levels that are achievable. This study also pointed out that, unlike chemotherapy drugs, Astaxanthin's abilities to reduce tumors cannot be due to toxicity. Even dietary concentrations as high as 2% did not induce toxicity in rats, mice or ferrets. The theory espoused by these researchers from the University of Minnesota's School of Medicine is that Astaxanthin's anti-tumor activity is related to its enhancement of the immune response (Jyonouchi, et al, 2000).

Other mice studies have also shown very promising results. One showed that Astaxanthin reduced the growth of transplanted breast tumors. This study tested Astaxanthin against two other carotenoids—beta carotene and canthaxanthin. The researchers found that "Mammary tumor growth inhibition by Astaxanthin was dose-dependent and was higher than that of canthaxanthin and beta carotene...Lipid peroxidation activity in tumors was lower ($P < 0.05$) in mice fed 0.4% astaxanthin, but not in those fed beta-carotene and canthaxanthin" (Chew, et al, 1999). The results showed that all three carotenoids had a positive effect, but that Astaxanthin worked best. (It is interesting to note that both of these carotenoids are present, along with lutein, in Natural Astaxanthin from Haematococcus algae, although the carotenoid complex is primarily Astaxanthin.) Another favorable study demonstrated that Astaxanthin suppressed spontaneous liver carcinogenesis (Nishino, et al, 1999). Further studies have shown that introduction of carcinogens such as benzopyrene to mice was positively affected when they were fed Astaxanthin; two specific types of cancer that appeared in the control group were inhibited in the Astaxanthin group (Lee, et al, 1997 and Lee, et al, 1998).

As we previously mentioned, Astaxanthin consumed in the diet reduced the incidence of tumor-promoting substances in the skin of hairless mice that were exposed to UVA and UVB radiation (Savoure, et al, 1995). Related research done at the Veterans Affairs Medical Center in Texas showed that Astaxanthin and beta carotene (but not lycopene) prevented UV-mediated carcinogenesis in mice (Black, H, 1998).

Astaxanthin, along with some other carotenoids, was found to be an effective anti-tumor agent in a series of studies on mice and rats at the Gifu University School of Medicine in Japan (Mori, et al, 1997). One of these studies found that Astaxanthin significantly reduced both the incidence and the proliferation of chemically-induced bladder cancer in mice. In this study, Astaxanthin was tested against canthaxanthin. It was found that the results with canthaxanthin were not statistically significant, while those with Astaxanthin were (Tanaka, et al, 1994). Two other studies showed the same effects in the oral cavity and the colon of rats; Astaxanthin reduced the incidence and the proliferation of cancers when carcinogenic chemicals were introduced (Tanaka, et al, 1995a and Tanaka, et al, 1995b). Lastly, a few different studies have shown Astaxanthin's positive effects on cancer of the liver in rats (Gradelet, et al, 1997, Gradelet, et al, 1998, Yang, et al, 1997 and Kurihara, et al, 2002).

What enables Astaxanthin to prevent cancer and shrink tumors? The three primary mechanisms of action can be any or all of these (Rousseau, et al, 1992):

1. Its potent biological antioxidant action
2. Its abilities as an immune system enhancer
3. Its action as a regulator of gene expression

In regards to regulating gene expression, basically, the cell to cell communication through the gap junctions is deficient in many human tumors. Improvement in this cell to cell communication tends to decrease tumor cell proliferation (Bertram, J, 1999). Astaxanthin is known to improve this intercellular communication.

There are several additional mechanisms that have been offered for Astaxanthin's anticarcinogenic effects. These include:

- Regulatory effects of Astaxanthin on transglutaminases (Savoure, et al, 1995)
- Inhibitory effect of Astaxanthin on metabolic activation of mutagens in bacteria (Rauscher, et al, 1998)
- Induction of apoptosis by Astaxanthin in mammary tumor cells (Kim, et al, 2001)
- Inhibition of the enzyme 5a-reductase (Anderson, M., 2001)
- Selective inhibition of DNA polymerases (Murakami, et al, 2002)
- Direct blocking of nitric oxide synthase (Ohgami, et al, 2003)

This is very technical information that scientists research to demonstrate how something works. Many products may have some benefit without the exact mechanism of action being known; in the case of Astaxanthin and its benefits in preventing carcinogenesis and shrinking tumors in animals, there are many different known mechanisms. Although this is very promising research, it remains to be seen if these same benefits will hold true in humans.

Help for Diabetics

Similar to the work with cancer, the research to date in the area of diabetes has not been tested in humans. It stands to reason that, since silent inflammation can cause diabetes, and since Astaxanthin can help reduce silent inflammation, that the use of Astaxanthin should have some benefit in people with diabetes and/or in preventing diabetes. We'll have to wait to prove this in human clinicals, but in the meantime there has been some very encouraging work in rodent models.

The four studies we'll analyze all took place in Japan at the Kyoto University of Medicine and at the Institute of Natural Medicine. The first study examined a special type of mice that are diabetic and obese, a generally accepted model for type-2 diabetic humans. Results demonstrated that Astaxanthin significantly reduced the blood glucose level of these mice. It further showed that the Astaxanthin treated group maintained their ability to secret insulin, and concluded: "These results indicate that astaxanthin can exert beneficial effects in diabetes, with preservation of beta-cell function" (Uchiyama, et al, 2002).

Diabetes adversely affects many different organs of the body. In particular, diabetes can cause the kidneys to malfunction, causing a condition called "nephropathy." This second study used the same diabetic, obese mice to examine how Astaxanthin could benefit the kidneys. The results: "After 12 weeks of treatment, the astaxanthin-treated group showed lower blood glucose compared with the non-treated group...treatment with astaxanthin ameliorated the progression and acceleration of diabetic nephropathy in the rodent model of type 2 diabetes. The results suggested that the antioxidant activity of astaxanthin reduced the oxidative stress on the kidneys and prevented renal cell damage. In conclusion, administration of astaxanthin might be a novel approach for the prevention of diabetic nephropathy" (Naito, et al, 2004).

The third study that touched on diabetes was previously cited in the section on cardiovascular benefits. This study in rats showed that after 22 weeks, Astaxanthin reduced blood pressure and improved cholesterol and triglyceride profiles, but it also showed a reduction in blood glucose levels. A significant reduction in fasting blood glucose levels as well as insulin resistance was noted, along with improvement in insulin sensitivity. A fascinating notation was made that Astaxanthin actually decreased the size of fat cells. "These results suggest that astaxanthin ameliorates insulin resistance by mechanisms involving the increase of glucose uptake, and by modulating the level of circulating lipid metabolites and adiponectin" (Hussein, et al, 2006).

Lastly, a recent study in diabetic mice showed that expression levels of genes extracted from the kidneys were decreased by Astaxanthin. This research may lead to a "better understanding of the genes and pathways involved in the anti-diabetic mechanism of astaxanthin" (Naito, et al, 2006).

Trying to Have a Baby? Give your Husband Natural Astaxanthin!

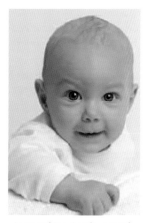

Astaxanthin: A safe, natural way to increase fertility

One of Natural Astaxanthin's most amazing attributes is its ability to help couples conceive. In the 1990's, a company in Sweden called AstaCarotene sponsored studies of the ability of Natural Astaxanthin to improve conception in pigs and horses. They did some experiments in which they fed the male animals Natural Astaxanthin and found that they would get a higher pregnancy rate, more offspring per female and more live births per female than in animals fed the same diet without Natural Astaxanthin. The logical conclusion was that Natural Astaxanthin somehow worked to make the males' sperm more potent (Lignell and Inboor, 2000). Fish and shrimp breeders have found similar benefits for breeding in marine species.

Researchers have recently taken the next logical step and tested Natural Astaxanthin (as AstaCarox® by AstaCarotene) in human couples that wanted babies but couldn't conceive. They took twenty couples that were trying to conceive for a minimum of at least twelve months. In each of these couples, the man was diagnosed as having abnormally poor semen quality. After three months of daily supplementation of a high dose of 16 mg per day of Natural Astaxanthin, five out of ten couples conceived! The researchers measured for oxidation of the semen: They found that reactive oxygen species decreased in the treatment group's semen. They also found that sperm motility, velocity and morphology improved for the men taking Astaxanthin (Comhaire and Mahmoud, 2003, and Comhaire, et al, 2005). Another study showing similar results was done previously. In this study the researchers concluded that supplementation with Natural Astaxanthin improved the quality of the spermatozoa, which is suggested to be the plausible explanation for the increased frequency of conception (Garem et al, 2002). It's incredible to think that the answer to many infertile couples' dreams of having children may be as easy as taking a few Natural Astaxanthin capsules each day, rather than going through different therapies that are very expensive and may still not yield the desired result. Imagine the stress and expense that could be saved by simply trying this natural remedy first.

Additional Research

Below are some very short synopses of several other studies that may have some relevance for future investigations into the benefits of Natural Astaxanthin in human nutrition. This is very preliminary research, but will probably lead to further investigation and human clinical trials.

A very promising study was done to see if there are possible benefits for **prostate problems** through the use of Astaxanthin. The inhibition of 5a-reductase has shown promise in treating the symptoms of **benign prostate hyperplasia,** and also as a possible means to **prevent or help treat prostate cancer.** Some in-vitro work was done which showed that Astaxanthin **inhibited 5a-reductase by 98%.** The researchers also took saw palmetto berry extract (which has also been reported to decrease the symptoms of benign prostate hyperplasia) and combined it with Astaxanthin, and found that the mixture showed a 20% greater inhibition of 5a-reductase than the saw palmetto extract alone. Lastly, they took prostate cancer cells and exposed them to Astaxanthin for nine days, after which they saw a 24% - 38% decrease in growth at different concentration levels (Anderson, M, 2004). These promising results indicate that Astaxanthin may be a potent soldier in the war on prostate cancer.

Recently, Dr. Chew from Washington State University, who had previously studied the anti-carcinogenic and immune enhancing properties of Natural Astaxanthin, did some new work in regards to Astaxanthin and DNA. Dr. Chew has since applied for a patent based on this promising research. It was found that Astaxanthin has an ability to **protect against DNA damage.** This property Astaxanthin has of protecting against DNA damage is directly related to its antioxidant capabilities. Dr. Chew and his colleague Dr. Park demonstrated that Natural Astaxanthin could prevent oxidative damage to DNA. What is very interesting is the dosage levels that they found to be effective. At dosage levels as low as 2 mg per day for four weeks, Drs. Chew and Park found that they could reduce oxidative damage to DNA by 40% (Chew, B, and Park, J, 2006). This is another example of just how powerful Natural Astaxanthin really is: At a dose that is one half the 4 mg capsule that is normally sold, **DNA damage can be reduced by 40%!**

A pre-clinical study was done in mice to test the ability of Astaxanthin and beta carotene to **prevent enlargement of the lymph nodes and reduce excess protein in the urine.** It was found that Astaxanthin significantly delayed the onset of both of these symptoms (which are associated with certain forms of cancer), and that Astaxanthin exerted more significant preventative action than beta carotene (Tomita, et al, 1993).

In another interesting pre-clinical study, Astaxanthin showed a positive effect on live births of baby minks. It was found that Astaxanthin given to the mothers significantly **reduced the number of stillborn births** (Hansen, et al, 2001).

Lastly, in-vitro work to explore a novel approach for the treatment of **asthma** showed favorable results with Astaxanthin. The researchers combined Astaxanthin with ginkgolide B and found that the combination **suppressed T-cell activation to a comparable level as two commonly sold anti-histamines** (Mahmoud, et al, 2004).

CHAPTER 8

Love your Pet?
Give it Natural Astaxanthin.

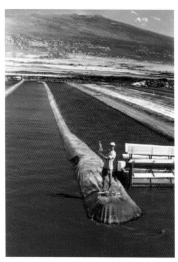

Think that Natural Astaxanthin is only good for humans? Think again—it's actually a wonderful supplement for your pet as well as an extraordinary feed ingredient for commercially grown livestock and farmed marine species. In fact, the use of Astaxanthin in farmed animals is a $200 - $300 million per year business. Unfortunately, most farmers use the vastly inferior synthetic Astaxanthin (which we'll discuss in more detail in Chapter 9) because it's less expensive. And to be honest, the main reason they use Astaxanthin is for coloring the flesh of fish. But there are also tremendous health benefits from using Astaxanthin that these farmers enjoy. And some of the smarter farmers are starting to use Natural Astaxanthin for their farmed animals based on compelling evidence that it is vastly superior to synthetic and phaffia-derived Astaxanthin sources.

Aquaculture can be raising fish in ponds or growing Haematococcus microalgae to make Natural Astaxanthin (above)

Uses of Astaxanthin in Aquaculture

For those of you who are not familiar with the term "aquaculture," it is basically farming in water. Growing the microalgae Haematococcus in ponds to make Natural Astaxanthin is one form of aquaculture.

The more common form is growing fish and shellfish in closed areas. As our world becomes more populated, and as the sustainability of fishing the Earth's oceans becomes doubtful, aquaculture appears to be a very attractive alternative. But there is a problem in raising certain species of fish and crustaceans in a closed environment—the normal diet of these species, which includes microalgae and/or krill, is substituted with commercial feeds. There is something missing from the natural food chain diet when raising marine animals on farms: Commercial feeds do not have the natural carotenoids present that are found in microalgae and krill. Due to the lack of carotenoids, many species of farmed fish or crustaceans will not have their natural color. This is a particular problem with aquacultured salmon and trout—without the addition of Astaxanthin to their diets, their flesh will appear beige or grayish. Unfortunately, consumers' appetites will not be whetted by this unnatural, bland looking fish.

So the main reason that many aquacultured species are given Astaxanthin in their diets is cosmetic—put simply, farmers want their fish to look appetizing so that people will buy them. But there is another reason that they use Astaxanthin that is much more relevant to our purposes in this book: Astaxanthin is an **essential nutrient** for many species of fish and crustaceans. It is basically a "vitamin" for some species—without Astaxanthin these animals' health will be severely compromised.

The essential nature of Astaxanthin for certain species has been demonstrated in different feed trials. One such trial is a perfect example: A study of the effects of Astaxanthin on **survival and growth rates** for Atlantic salmon fry; they found that without Astaxanthin, only 17% of these tiny fish survived to become adult fish. As the researchers increased the amount of Astaxanthin in the diet from 0.4 parts per million (ppm), to 1.0 ppm and finally up to 13.7 ppm, the percentage of fry that survived increased. In fact, by the time they went from zero up to 1.0 ppm, **the amount of fish that survived increased from 17% all the way up to 87%!** And when they reached the maximum levels used in this study of 13.7 ppm, the survival rate increased to over 98%! (If this isn't proof that Astaxanthin is an essential nutrient for salmon, then nothing is.)

This study went on to examine Astaxanthin's effect on the **growth rate** in these salmon. A similar effect to that of the survival rate was found: At zero Astaxanthin inclusion, the fry grew very slowly; when the feed reached 1.0 ppm Astaxanthin, the fry were growing more than twice as fast; and by the time the feed reached the maximum value tested of 13.7 ppm Astaxanthin, the fry **grew over six times faster than the fish given no Astaxanthin**. It's really amazing to think about how far a little Astaxanthin goes—13.7 ppm is a very small amount, and 1.0 ppm is practically nothing. Yet even at the 1.0 ppm level fish grow twice as fast and 70% more fish survive! You can see that pigmenting the salmon's flesh is not the only reason why salmon farmers make sure their feed contains Astaxanthin—the pigmentation is simply what enables them to sell the fish. They're also using Astaxanthin to keep the young fish alive and to make them grow much faster, two things that help ensure the economic viability of any farming operation.

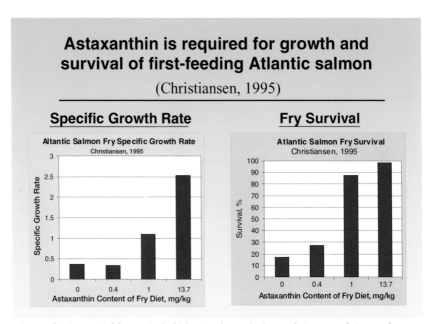

Astaxanthin is essential for survival of Atlantic salmon. It also vastly improves their growth rate.

And growth and survival are only two of the proven health benefits for aquacultured species. Others benefits include **improved breeding and egg quality, improved stress resistance, improved immunity to diseases and even better feed conversion ratios** (the amount of feed needed for a specific weight gain). In one experiment done with sturgeon in Russia, the **feed conversion ratio improved by 30%** (Ilyasov and Golovin, 2003). And both sturgeon and rainbow trout have been shown to have **increased immunity** due to elevated humoral factors (Luzzano, et al, 2003 and Ilyasov and Golovin, 2003). In Japan, Natural Astaxanthin was found to **increase both the quantity of eggs as well as the**

quality of the eggs (Watanabe, et al, 2003 and Aquis, et al, 2001). And inclusion of 10 ppm in red sea bream and striped jack broodstock **increased the number of eggs produced by three times** (Watanabe, et al, 2003). Additionally, the ability of Astaxanthin to help with **stress resistance** is well documented. In several studies, tiger prawns have been shown to be much more resistant to three different types of induced stress when fed Natural Astaxanthin. In fact, these studies also showed an interesting difference between Astaxanthin sources: Natural Astaxanthin was found to work considerably better than synthetic (Darachai, et al, 1999).

When comparing natural to synthetic Astaxanthin sources, it's not only in stress resistance where natural comes out on top. You may remember from Chapter 2 that Natural Astaxanthin from microalgae was proven to be over twenty times stronger than synthetic in an antioxidant test of free radical elimination (Bagchi, 2001). The natural variety of Astaxanthin also has clear functional advantages in fish and shellfish over the synthetic and phaffia yeast-derived varieties. In one study in shrimp, Natural Astaxanthin was considerably better than synthetic in increasing both survival and growth rates (Darachai, et al, 1998). And because natural Astaxanthin is esterified and has a different shape than the free Astaxanthin found in the other forms, it is able to more easily reach throughout the entire body. For example, Natural Astaxanthin is able to get into the skin of species such as sea bream and many tropical fish better, consequently bringing out more vibrant and natural-looking color in their skin.

There are many other far-ranging benefits for Astaxanthin in aquaculture. Some of them seem trivial (in one study, it was found that Astaxanthin **decreased**

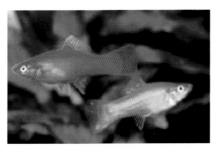

Two of the same species of fish, the top was fed Natural Astaxanthin and the bottom was not. Note the deeper, more vibrant color and healthier look of the Natural Astaxanthin-fed fish.

the incidence of cataracts in salmon (Waagbo, et al, 2003). People eating salmon may not care if the fish had cataracts, but it is just one more indication of Astaxanthin's many health benefits in animals). In any event, if you want to have healthy fish in your fish tank at home and you want them to live a long life, you should certainly give them some Natural Astaxanthin.

A Wonderful Reward for "Man's Best Friend"

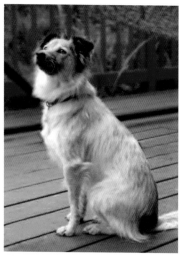

Astaxanthin can help keep your dog healthy and active

While tropical fish are a fairly popular pet, dogs and other mammals are on the top of most people's lists. We've seen countless references to mouse and rat studies in which Astaxanthin helped improve various facets of their health. Most of these benefits should also be found in other mammals, including humans, although to be completely certain, studies would have to be done on each species. There has been some promising work done with many different species. One of the most exciting species that seems to thrive when given Natural Astaxanthin is also one of the most common household pets, the dog.

Some of the first dog owners to start feeding their dogs Natural Astaxanthin were the sled doggers in Alaska. Before any experiments had been done, these very competitive dog owners were finding that, as with human athletes, Astaxanthin is a secret weapon for dogs too. The premise behind the sled doggers' use of Astaxanthin is quite simple: Aerobic exercise is a source of harmful oxidation in the body caused by reactive oxygen species (ROS). These ROS can quickly consume the available antioxidants in an athlete's body. As a result athletes need to ingest far more antioxidants in order for their bodies to respond well to the ROS produced, and to maintain a healthy oxidative state within the body during exercise. We looked at this progression closely in Chapter 6.

It appears that what's true for "man" is also true for "man's best friend." Sled dogs work is grueling and they spend extended amounts of time in harsh conditions when pulling sleds; therefore, you can be sure that the ROS in their bodies are at a peak. So what better way to control these oxidants in the dogs' bodies than by giving them the world's strongest natural antioxidant?

A study published in 2000 evaluated the effects of dietary supplementation with various carotenoids on sled dogs. This study found that dietary supplementation with carotenoids resulted in increased plasma concentrations of antioxidants. DNA oxidation was decreased and resistance of lipoprotein particles to in-vitro oxidation was increased. They concluded, "Antioxidant supplementation of sled dogs may attenuate exercise-induced oxidative damage" (Baskin, et al, 2000).

In the May/June 2006 issue of the sled doggers' favorite publication, Mushing Magazine, there was an article on nutrition for sled dogs. This article was an interview with a well known nutritionist and sled dog open class racer, Dr. Arleigh Reynolds, PhD. In this article, Dr. Reynolds speaks about Astaxanthin specifically: "It is one of the few things that I have studied that not only shows

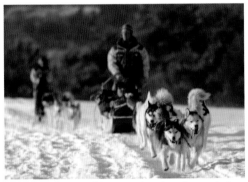

measurable improvement in blood parameters but also visibly improves the dog's performance."

In other research, a company that we mentioned in Chapter 7 did an experiment in dogs with excellent results. The company, Cardax, used their patented injectable Astaxanthin to see if it would have benefits for the dogs' hearts. They had previously demonstrated this in mice, but felt that the canine model is more relevant as an

Just like salmon and humans, dogs benefit greatly from Natural Astaxanthin's superior antioxidant activity.

indication of potential benefits in humans. They were successful—their study demonstrated that Astaxanthin had "**marked cardioprotective properties in both rodents and canines.**" They concluded that, based on the excellent performance in dogs, this injectable Astaxanthin may be a means to **prevent heart damage from myocardial injury**, and may be useful in angioplasty, stenting and coronary bypass surgery (Gross and Lockwood, 2005).

While there certainly is not a mass of scientific experiments investigating the benefits of Astaxanthin in dogs, there are some positive studies as well as anecdotal evidence. Also, logical extensions of existing information from other species indicate that Astaxanthin should work like magic for dogs. As a respected nutritionist and scientist, Dr. Reynolds sees it in his sled dogs' blood. And as an avid sled dogger, he also visibly sees it in their performance. There is now enough evidence of Astaxanthin's benefits in dogs that some of the world's largest pet food manufacturers have begun to investigate Astaxanthin in self-funded studies. In fact, there is already a patent that has been issued to a large pet food manufacturer regarding the use of Astaxanthin in dogs. Soon, you'll probably be able to buy dog food with Astaxanthin already mixed in it; but you don't have to wait for a pet food company to do this for you—you can buy some gelcaps yourself and mix one in with your dog's food each day.

Any Animal Will Benefit from Natural Astaxanthin

Mice and rats, fish and shrimp, and even dogs have demonstrated health benefits from Astaxanthin in the studies we've already cited. We've seen an abundance of animal studies showing that Astaxanthin **improves immunity, supports cardiovascular health, increases endurance, brings antioxidant protection to the eyes and brain, and even reduces tumors and prevents cancer** in different laboratory animals. But this research was mostly in mice and rats. What about other animals? Can cats, horses, parrots and snakes obtain advantages from ingesting Astaxanthin as well? Although there is not scientific evidence for every species, the overwhelming indication is that all animals should benefit from this wonderful substance.

There is another commercial use in animals now besides aquaculture, tropical fish and sled dog feeds. Natural Astaxanthin is also used by a few chicken feed manufacturers. Again, as with salmon, the main reason is to pigment the egg yolks a deep, rich color.

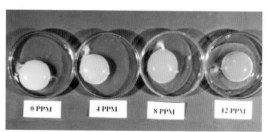

A little goes a long way: Egg yolks go from yellow to a deep orange with only 4–8 parts per million of Natural Astaxanthin.

But just as with the salmon farmers, you can be sure that the chicken farmers are deriving plenty of health benefits from feeding their chickens Astaxanthin. One very interesting study examined the effects Astaxanthin had when given to layer hens. It was found that Astaxanthin **decreased the overall mortality of the chickens, increased their fertility and improved their overall health status**. In addition, **egg production increased while salmonella infections decreased dramatically**, which was probably due to a stronger membrane formation. A US patent was issued for this groundbreaking work in poultry (Lignell, et al, 1998).

There has been some research concerning Astaxanthin's effects in other animals as well. We'll briefly look at a few different studies, which you'll see are quite varied. The first was a **study done with horses for a life threatening disease** call equine exertional rhabdomyolysis. This is an acute disease that is potentially fatal. It manifests in the destruction of muscle which occurs because of a shortage of oxygen transporting to the muscles and a lack of protein storage in the muscles. This affliction can end the career or even kill a thoroughbred race horse in its prime. A very positive study was done on eight race horses with this horrible disease. They were supplemented with 30 mg of Astaxanthin per day, and **after only two to three weeks the animals were symptom-free and able to**

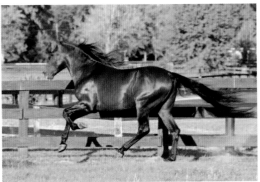

continue training and racing! When the dosage was reduced or supplementation ceased, the symptoms returned after approximately two weeks. The researcher was awarded a US patent for his outstanding work (Lignell, A, 2001).

The same researcher, Ake Lignell of Sweden received a third patent for his innovative work in animals. He examined the effect that

Astaxanthin completely cured a life threatening muscle disease in race horses

Natural Astaxanthin has on **breeding and fertility** in livestock animals. Just as he had discovered in his groundbreaking work with chickens in 1998, Dr. Lignell discovered that Astaxanthin **increased the fertility of pigs, cattle and sheep**. For example, in pigs, the research showed that Astaxanthin significantly **improved three separate markers of fertility: The birth rate, the percentage of live births and the number of pigs born per sow** (Lignell and Inboor, 2000).

There is a wide range of other evidence of Astaxanthin's benefits in mammals. In Chapter 4 we saw how Astaxanthin can help **protect the lens of a pig's eye against oxidative damage** in-vitro (Wu, et al, 2006). A study of hyperlipidemic rabbits found that Astaxanthin was superior to Vitamin E in helping to **stabilize plaque in the arteries, and concluded that it could be useful in the fight**

against atherosclerosis (Li, et al, 2004). Another study in rabbits showed that red yeast rice and policosanol helped to protect the heart's aortic wall. The researchers then found that by adding Astaxanthin to the mix, the effect was far superior; when adding Astaxanthin the **lipid infiltration into the aortic wall was almost completely prevented** (Setnikar, et al, 2005). Another study that looked at health and reproduction in minks found that Astaxanthin showed a positive effect on live births of baby minks. It was documented that Astaxanthin given to the mothers significantly **reduced the number of stillborn births** (Hansen, et al, 2001).

In conclusion, so that readers can decide for themselves if it's prudent to give Astaxanthin to their pets, let's review all of its potential benefits in animals as evidenced from the studies we've cited:

• Prevents cancer	• Protects the eyes and brain
• Reduces tumor size	• Decreases pain
• Promotes cardiovascular health	• Increases endurance
• Improves immunity	• Improves fertility
• Prevents diabetes	• Reduces stillborn deaths
• Increases stress resistance	• Prevents DNA damage
• Inhibits H. pylori bacteria	• Prevents cell membrane damage
• Reduces gastric ulcerations	• Prevents enlargement of lymph nodes
• Aids the liver in detoxification	• Improves growth rate in young animals
• Prevents cataracts	• Improves survival rate

Granted, some of the work cited is from preliminary studies and further research is needed, but with this exhaustive list of potential benefits, pet owners should be giving Natural Astaxanthin to their pets every day. (As well as taking it themselves!)

CHAPTER 9

Other Vital Information

There is a great deal of information about Natural Astaxanthin that does not fit nicely into any of the preceding chapters, but is nonetheless important for the reader to know. Such topics include safety, dosage information, differences between various sources of Astaxanthin and between different manufacturers, as well as an examination of some of the problems in marketing Astaxanthin such as stability issues and accurate measurement of Natural Astaxanthin.

Safety

Natural Astaxanthin has been consumed in the diet for as long as humans have eaten anything red or pink from the sea. For example, the equivalent amount of one 4 mg capsule of Natural Astaxanthin can be found in a four ounce (100 gram) serving of sockeye salmon, the salmon species that has by far the highest Astaxanthin concentration. It is interesting to note that there are huge differences in the Astaxanthin concentrations between various species of salmon. For instance, you would have to eat two pounds or almost one kilogram of Atlantic salmon, the species that has the lowest Astaxanthin concentration, in order to get the equivalent of one 4 mg capsule serving (Turujman, et al, 1997).

It is refreshing to know that for as long as Natural Astaxanthin has been consumed, there has never been an indication of toxicity, negative interaction with any drug, supplement or food, or any other contraindication. And in the ten years that Natural Astaxanthin has been sold as a dietary supplement, there has not been any documented adverse incident, not even an allergic reaction. This information is contrary to the case with other commercial sources of Astaxanthin, such as the Astaxanthin that is chemically synthesized from petrochemicals or the Astaxanthin that is grown on mutated yeast. "Natural Astaxanthin from Haematococcus microalgae has never been associated with any toxicity in the reported literature or in field studies, and numerous animal and human studies lend support to its safety" (Dore, J, 2002 and Maher, T, 2000).

Haematococcus was first reviewed by the US Food and Drug Administration as the trademarked supplement BioAstin® in 1999 (Docket No. 95S-0316) and cleared for marketing as a dietary ingredient. It has also been approved by the US government for aquaculture applications. This approval of Haematococcus-derived Astaxanthin has taken place in many other countries for both humans and animals, including the European Union and Japan.

As previously discussed, the highest concentration of Natural Astaxanthin in the human diet is found in salmon. There is a tremendous range of Astaxanthin concentrations in salmon flesh, from 1-58 mg/kg. The results from a study on salmon Astaxanthin levels is below (Turujman, et al, 1997):

Species	Astaxanthin Range	Astaxanthin Average
Wild sockeye salmon	30-58 mg/kg	40.4 mg/kg
Wild Coho salmon	9-28 mg/kg	13.8 mg/kg
Wild pink salmon	3-7 mg/kg	5.4 mg/kg
Wild chum salmon	1-8 mg/kg	5.6 mg/kg
Wild Chinook king salmon	1-22 mg/kg	8.9 mg/kg
Wild Atlantic salmon	5-7 mg/kg	5.3 mg/kg
Average of all species		**13.2 mg/kg**

The average Astaxanthin concentration ranges from 5.3 mg/kg in Atlantic salmon to 40.4 mg/kg in sockeye salmon. The average of all species was calculated to be 13.2 mg/kg. Since the average human would consume about 0.25 kg of fish flesh in one meal, this results in the lowest intake of 1.3 mg of Astaxanthin from Atlantic salmon, 3.3 mg of Astaxanthin from "average" salmon and 10.1 mg of Astaxanthin from sockeye salmon. This corresponds to the range of dosages for various commercial Astaxanthin offerings.

Other natural carotenoid pigments are found in Haematococcus-derived Astaxanthin including canthaxanthin, lutein and beta carotene, but they are present at roughly 5% of the level of Astaxanthin. These carotenoids are commonly found in fruits and vegetables in the normal human diet. Total canthaxanthin, lutein and beta carotene intake from a common dose of a Natural Astaxanthin supplement would be less than 0.25 mg/day. Canthaxanthin is currently allowed for use in coloring foods under the US Code of Federal Regulations (CFR 21 section 73.75) at levels not to exceed 30 mg per pound of food or pint of beverage. Thus, the canthaxanthin ingested from a normal dose of a Natural Astaxanthin supplement is over 100-fold less than would be ingested from a pound of food or pint of liquid colored with the maximum allowance for canthaxanthin. The usual recommended doses of beta carotene and lutein are 20-60 mg/day and 3-6 mg/day, respectively, which are ten times to over 200 times the amounts in a normal daily serving of a Haematococcus-based Astaxanthin supplement.

Many human safety studies in addition to all the human clinical trials and all the animal trials have never shown any adverse effects for Astaxanthin. In addition, extensive acute toxicity work in mice and rats has been completed, including studies where the rodents were fed tremendous doses in comparison with their body weight. In each of these, no mortality or symptoms of toxicity were reported. Additionally, safety research has been completed on many other animal species. In one of these studies, mega-doses fed to pregnant rabbits resulted in no adverse events to either the mothers or the fetuses. (Extensive safety information can be found at www.cyanotech.com or by contacting the Publisher at 808.326.1353.)

Stability

Most of Natural Astaxanthin's many diverse benefits in human nutrition are in some way related to its supreme antioxidant power. This inherently poses a problem for the manufacturer and the consumer: For the manufacturer, great care must be taken to ensure that the Natural Astaxanthin does not oxidize during processing, handling, encapsulating or tableting, and finally during packaging and storage. For the consumer, the problem is making sure that you purchase an Astaxanthin supplement that has the full amount of Astaxanthin in the pill that is stated on the label. This is even more complicated because, as we'll see later in this chapter, some manufacturers do not even know how to accurately measure Astaxanthin, which actually involves some very complicated lab work.

Astaxanthin is exceptionally unstable when subjected to oxygen. Because it is such a strong antioxidant, the Astaxanthin molecule will begin to bond with oxygen molecules in the air. Once it oxidizes, it will break down into a degradation product called "astacene" that has no benefit to humans or animals. Extreme care must be taken when handling Astaxanthin to be sure that it does not oxidize.

The process used to extract the concentrated oil containing Astaxanthin and the supporting carotenoids from the Haematococcus microalgae is another very important step. There are several different ways to extract Natural Astaxanthin from Haematococcus. The state-of-the-art manner is to use a super-critical, solvent-free extraction at high pressure which uses only carbon dioxide. Not only does this prevent any unwanted solvent residue, but this also provides for a more stable Astaxanthin oil product.

Delivery Methods

The next step in the process is finding a suitable delivery method to get the Astaxanthin into the body. The most common method is in a gelatin capsule. Gelcaps can provide protection from oxygen for an oil-based Astaxanthin product. But not all gelcaps are created equal; it is important that a quality manufacturer is used. And particular care must be exercised when moving into a vegetarian gelcap, as many do not properly protect the Astaxanthin within. If you take Astaxanthin in a poor quality capsule, it won't become a safety issue; but what can happen is that some or all of the Astaxanthin can oxidize into the inert degradation product astacene, so you won't get the benefits you're looking for.

Even worse than the problems with capsules are the problems with Astaxanthin in powder form. Powdered nutraceutical ingredients are used for making tablets or for putting products into hard-shell capsules. Most powders containing Astaxanthin are extremely unstable. The only way to ensure stability is to microencapsulate the powder into tiny gelatin beads, each so small that the finished product looks like a powder. As with the gelcaps, it is imperative that this is done by a quality manufacturer with the expertise to successfully protect the fragile Astaxanthin molecules from air. As of the writing of this book, there are only a handful of manufacturers in the world that are capable of doing this, and it remains a very technical (and expensive)

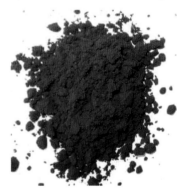

Astaxanthin powder that has not been microencapsulated. This product will not be stable and should not be used for consumer products.

process. But it is an imperative step in order to protect a fragile substance like Astaxanthin.

It is a very frightening fact that there are products sold commercially that do not come anywhere close to maintaining sufficient stability. Some Astaxanthin products bought off the shelf and tested have shown Astaxanthin levels at less than half the label claim! Be very careful when choosing brands and only go with a respected manufacturer.

Other potential delivery methods include functional foods and energy or sports drinks. As Astaxanthin is a relatively new product, there have not been many product offerings in this area yet, although there will most likely be a trend toward these novel delivery methods in the future. One very unique delivery method as a functional food already being employed is in the eggs you see below. These eggs come from Sweden; the name "Kronaggs Guldgula" translates in English to "Crown Eggs, Golden Yolk." This company feeds their chickens Natural Astaxanthin, so that their eggs contain Astaxanthin. The people eating these eggs, in turn, are consuming Astaxanthin in their diets.

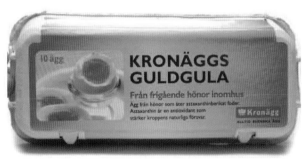

*Unique functional food—An egg with Natural Astaxanthin!
Look at the color of the yolk—dark and rich because of Astaxanthin.*

The Kronagg company uses Natural Astaxanthin for a few reasons: First of all, they've taken a product—eggs—that has become pretty much a commodity, and effectively distinguished themselves from their competition. In order to do this, they give infomation about Astaxanthin on the front of the carton. (While most people reading this book cannot read Swedish, one can easily make out the words "Astaxanthin" and "antioxidant" on the label. It is interesting to note that once the egg carton is opened, there is a great deal of additional information on the inside lid telling the consumer about the benefits of Astaxanthin in much greater detail.)

So, Kronagg has wisely distinguished themselves from all their competitors by making a "new and improved" egg. They point out that these eggs are better than other eggs because they contain a strong antioxidant. Their eggs are also different in that the intense pigment in Natural Astaxanthin gives the egg yolks a deep, golden color. (As we saw in the chapter on uses for animals, a very small addition of Astaxanthin to the chicken feed will significantly alter the color of the egg yolks.) Kronagg sells their eggs for a slightly higher price than their competitors, but they have still managed to capture a significant percentage of the Swedish egg market in a relatively short time because many consumers want a superior egg.

Dosage and Bioavailability

Several studies have validated Astaxanthin's bioavailability. Many animal models have found Astaxanthin throughout the bodies of rodents while human studies measuring blood levels of Astaxanthin have proven that this carotenoid is absorbed by humans through oral consumption (Osterlie, et al, 2000 and Mercke, et al, 2003). But we have to look closely at a number of factors to understand the correct dosage level for humans.

The dosage levels in human clinical trials have ranged from as low as 2 mg per day in positive immunity trials, to as high 16 mg per day in the intriguing male fertility trials. Other trials have been everywhere in between. What exact dosage is the proper one for most people?

The answer to this question depends on a few things: First of all, for what purpose are you using Astaxanthin? Secondly, are you a 5% absorber or a 90% absorber?

Let's talk about the second question first: Different humans have a wide ranging ability to absorb carotenoids. For example, your body might be able to absorb 90% of the carotenoids you eat, while your friend (or even a close relative) may only be able to absorb 5%. This makes it difficult to recommend a specific dosage for all people. If your body absorbs 90% of carotenoids and you take only 1 mg of Astaxanthin, you'll get the same benefit as your friend (who absorbs 5% of carotenoids) when he or she takes 18 mg! This huge disparity makes it difficult for supplement manufacturers to decide what dosage to recommend on their labels.

The other key question is why you're taking Astaxanthin. If you're a man taking it who's been diagnosed with poor semen quality and you and your wife want to have a baby, you probably should take the full level at which the fertility study was done — 16 mg per day. If you're just looking for an antioxidant and immune system boost and you're already eating a good diet, you might get by with only 2 mg per day.

A major factor that determines how well people will absorb Natural Astaxanthin is when it is taken: It is highly recommended that Natural Astaxanthin supplements are taken with meals, preferably with a meal that has some fat content. This is similar to other carotenoids, all of which are fat soluble. These lipophilic ("fat-loving") nutrients, taken in the absence of fats, are poorly absorbed; when taken with fats, the absorption is maximized. One study centered around this premise tested the bioavailability of Natural Astaxanthin in three different lipid-based formulas, all of which resulted in better absorption than a formula that did not have any additional lipids (Mercke, et al, 2003). The message is clear—be sure to take your Astaxanthin with fats, or at the very least in a gelcap containing oil as a base, in order to maximize the benefits.

The recommended daily dosage amongst manufacturers has become fairly standardized at a 4 mg per day level for the average person who has no serious concerns (such as low fertility or severe joint or tendon problems). Following is a table of recommended dosages that is provided as a rough guideline for consumers.

Use	Recommended Dosage
Antioxidant	2 – 4 mg per day
Arthritis	4 – 12 mg per day
Tendonitis or Carpal Tunnel Syndrome	4 – 12 mg per day
Silent Inflammation (C-reactive protein)	4 – 12 mg per day
Internal Sunscreen	4 – 8 mg per day
Internal Beauty and Skin Improvement	2 – 4 mg per day
Immune System Enhancer	2 – 4 mg per day
Cardiovascular Health	4 – 8 mg per day
Strength and Endurance	4 – 8 mg per day
Brain and Central Nervous System Health	4 – 8 mg per day
Eye Health	4 – 8 mg per day
Topical Use	20 – 100 parts per million

When deciding what is the right level for yourself, we suggest you start with the lower dosage in the range, and then see what kind of results you have after a month. If you're not getting the desired results, increase your dosage. For most people, one 4 mg gelcap is just right, but there are people who need two or three gelcaps each day to get their desired results. Also, some people take the opposite approach: They start at a higher dose, say 8 mg per day for the first few weeks, at which point they can bring the dosage down to 4 mg per day. The important things to remember are that:

• There is no toxicity level, so taking more won't hurt you.
• Astaxanthin is so powerful that even a little bit in a multivitamin or an antioxidant formula will go a long way toward helping prevent all the life-threatening diseases associated with oxidation and inflammation.

Other Commercial Applications

There are a few other ways in which Natural Astaxanthin can be used that we haven't mentioned. Some of these are already being commercialized (such as in topical applications) and others are still in development. As time goes on, new applications will undoubtedly be found.

Natural Astaxanthin as a Food Color

Natural Astaxanthin is an intense pigment. A very small amount can lend a beautiful salmon hue to any product in which it can be suitably mixed. This leads to a logical question: Why not use Natural Astaxanthin as a food color?

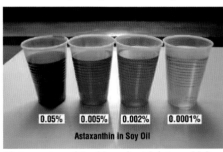

0.05%   0.005%   0.002%   0.0001%
Astaxanthin in Soy Oil

Photo courtesy of Food Ingredient Solutions, LLC, New York, NY

This is a great idea, and since there is a serious lack of natural red food colors from appropriate sources (the most popular natural red color today is made from dead beetles), we're sure to see this happening in the near future. One company has already started some research and development in this area. Note the various possible shades in the photo of Natural Astaxanthin in soybean oil.

And it's very interesting to note how little it takes to make a reddish hue. At 0.002% it's already quite reddish. When you get up to 0.05%, the red pigment is so intense that it almost looks black!

Cosmetic Applications

Antioxidants have outstanding benefits when used topically. Some leading cosmetic manufacturers use antioxidants in many different products. Vitamin E was one of the first antioxidants to be used topically, and is still probably the most widely used in topical products. But since Natural Astaxanthin is so much stronger than Vitamin E, it stands to reason that it would be a great addition to a variety of cosmetic products.

There's a question that is probably coming into many people's minds after seeing the dark, reddish-black color of the soybean oil at a concentration of only 0.05% above: No one would want a cosmetic product that is such a dark color. But that's the beauty of Natural Astaxanthin—it's so powerful that a little goes a very long way. At 550 times the antioxidant strength of Vitamin E, cosmetic manufacturers can use a small fraction of the amount of Natural Astaxanthin in a formula when compared to the amount they would use of Vitamin E—and still get a powerful antioxidant effect.

Many leading cosmetic manufacturers are already doing just that—using small amounts of Natural Astaxanthin in the 20 – 100 parts per million range. This gives the products a beautiful salmon hue, and it also gives them a great antioxidant benefit that should help the skin substantially. One of the most com-

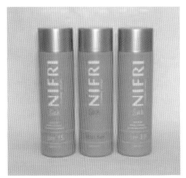

Nifri Sunscreen and After Sun Products. Distributed in Europe by OTC Pharma, The Netherlands.

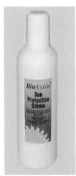

BioAstin Sun Protection Crème. Distributed in the United Kingdom by Life Long Products.

95

mon uses to date is in sunscreen products. In sunscreens, the benefits of Natural Astaxanthin are two-fold: First, it will help sunscreen to better protect the skin from sunburn and UV damage (Arakane, K, 2002). Secondly, the antioxidant properties will help repair previously damaged skin.

Not only are sunscreen manufacturers starting to astutely include Natural Astaxanthin in their sunscreens, but several cosmetic manufacturers are starting to use Natural Astaxanthin in various facial creams, body creams and lipsticks. Again, the Astaxanthin will help protect exposed skin from the sun and at the same time help to heal damaged skin.

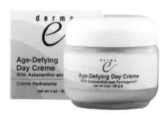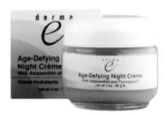

Samples of the derma e® fine line of Cosmetics Containing Natural Astaxanthin. Photos courtesy of derma e® Natural Bodycare, Simi Valley, CA.

Other Ideas

There are many other uses for Natural Astaxanthin that will be appearing in the coming years. We can only imagine all the novel uses that might be found for this powerful antioxidant, anti-inflammatory and natural red color. A good example of a novel use for Natural Astaxanthin involves the gums. There is a great deal of testimonial evidence that Natural Astaxanthin consumed internally can reduce or eliminate gum disease. In addition to the testimonial evidence, it is logical that a strong anti-inflammatory and antioxidant applied topically to the gums could reduce gum disease. There is already development work being done by a few toothpaste manufacturers to test the viability of a toothpaste with Natural Astaxanthin as a means for treating gum disease. Don't be surprised if you start seeing this marketed in a few years.

Differences between Cyanotech's Technology and Other Manufacturers

Now, let's look at the differences between manufacturers of Astaxanthin: Currently there are already a handful of manufacturers of Astaxanthin for human

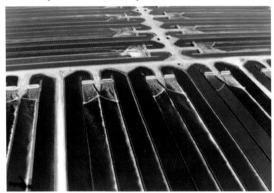

nutrition, all of which are from Haematococcus microalgae with the exception of one product from mutated Phaffia yeast. We'll see in the next section why this Phaffia yeast product as well as synthetic Astaxanthin are vastly inferior forms. In the meantime, let's examine the difference between manufac-

Overhead view of Spirulina ponds, Kona, Hawaii. Spirulina is a much easier microalgae species to grow than Haematococcus.

turers of Natural Astaxanthin from microalgae.

The complexities of growing and processing microalgae vary immensely according to the species. The most common species of microalgae produced and marketed for human consumption is a blue green algae called Spirulina (Arthrospira platensis). While there are great differences in quality between the different farms producing Spirulina around the world, the actual growing process is much easier than growing Haematococcus microalgae. This is because Spirulina grows in a very alkaline environment; growers must add large amounts of baking soda to get the alkalinity in the ponds up to about 10 on the pH scale. This also prevents other organisms from invading the ponds. Haematococcus poses a special challenge because it grows in a pH neutral environment. This is why there are only a few companies in the world that have been able to successfully produce this species. In fact, several companies have gone bankrupt trying to figure out how to successfully grow Haematococcus.

Cyanotech Corporation has been commercially producing microalgal products for 23 years. During this time, advanced technology has been developed which, combined with its location on the pristine Kona Coast of the Big Island of Hawaii, allows Cyanotech to produce uni-algal, contamination-free products.

97

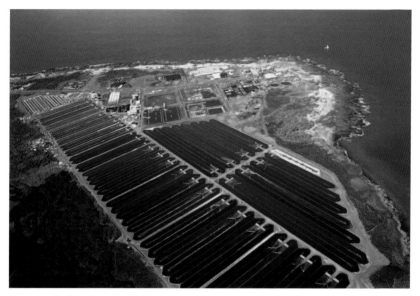
Cyanotech's 90 acre (40 hectare) microalgae farm on the pristine Kona Coast of Hawaii's Big Island

Cyanotech's most advanced technology is used for the production of Natural Astaxanthin from Haematococcus microalgae. The initial production of Haematococcus takes place in closed culture systems, some as large as 40,000 liters. This is followed by a short, five to seven day, "reddening" cycle conducted in 500,000 liter open culture ponds. At each stage of Astaxanthin production, Haematococcus cultures are closely monitored by microscopic examination to ensure the cultures are pure and free from contaminating organisms. After the reddening cycle, the Haematococcus cultures are harvested, washed and dried. The final step for the production of Astaxanthin is extraction of dried Haematococcus biomass using supercritical carbon dioxide to produce a purified oleoresin, absolutely free of any biological or environmental contamination. As we mentioned above, this supercritical extraction process is a vital step in ensuring the proper stability, potency, and purity of all Natural Astaxanthin products.

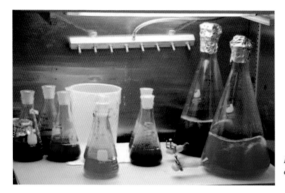

Haematococcus cultures in the experimental stage

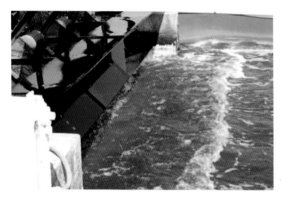

Haematococcus a few days away from harvest stage

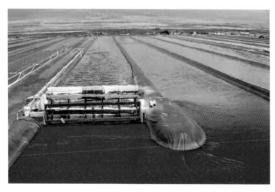

A Haematococcus pond ready for harvest

All other commercial producers of Haematococcus today currently use closed culture systems. Many falsely claim that fully closed systems are superior because they protect the algae from contamination. This is a misconception—that closed culture production of microalgal products eliminates contamination from unwanted organisms. Closed culture systems can be (and often are) contaminated by unwanted algae, fungi, and protozoa. When this does occur, elimination of the biological contamination in closed culture systems can be very difficult because of the high surface area and many "nooks and crannies" in such systems. Indeed, persistent contamination of closed cultures systems has led to serious problems for microalgae companies in California, Hawaii (not Cyanotech), and Europe—in all three cases it led to bankruptcy for these companies. Currently, a new Haematococcus production facility in Hawaii which uses small BioDomes has found that it is extremely difficult and expensive to control contamination. The economic viability of this facility is in question.

Cyanotech's closed culture systems, as well as its open pond systems, have been designed based on many years of experience to minimize these problems and to ensure production of contamination-free microalgal products. And the supercritical solvent free extraction that the algae go through before reaching the consumer fully ensures that the product is safe and pure. On top of all the testing during the growing phases and the supercritical extraction, each finished production lot of Natural Astaxanthin at Cyanotech is fully tested under meticulous quality control parameters in state-of-the-art laboratories.

Cyanotech's Natural Astaxanthin production is registered as an ISO 9001-2000 Quality Management System, and holds a Food Establishment Permit from the State of Hawaii Department of Health for manufacturing and processing. Cyanotech also uses current Good Manufacturing Practices (c-GMP) and operates under US Food and Drug Administration (FDA) guidelines. And as previously mentioned, each lot of Cyanotech's Natural Astaxanthin goes through rigorous quality control to ensure the highest quality and purity.

Furthermore, extensive stability testing is done to ensure that products will have the stated amount of Astaxanthin by the time they get to the consumer. This is a critical step in the process—it's not good enough to just produce Haematococcus—you have to make sure that the Astaxanthin is protected and stable throughout the growing process, the extraction, the encapsulation or tableting and the packaging, otherwise all the previous work will be in vain.

In addition to unsurpassed quality and purity, Cyanotech's many years of

experience and proprietary technology allow it to produce
of Natural Astaxanthin than its competitors and maintain a
half of the worldwide market for human nutrition Astaxanth   ...s. When
you purchase Astaxanthin, make sure it's from one of Cyanotech's many worldwide distributors.

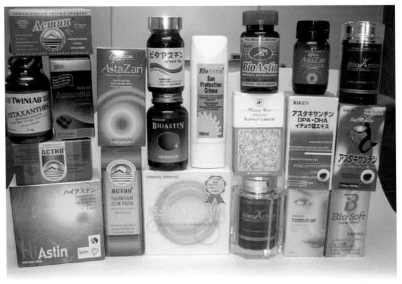

Just a few of the many consumer products from around the world featuring Cyanotech's
Natural Astaxanthin.

Natural versus Synthetic and Phaffia-Derived Astaxanthin

There are a few other sources of Astaxanthin besides the natural form from
Haematococcus microalgae that we have been devoting most of our attention to
so far in this book. The principal alternatives to microalgae-based Astaxanthin
may be commercially viable but are not nearly as practical and, except for the
case of eating wild salmon, are certainly not as health-giving as taking
Astaxanthin from Haematococcus microalgae in capsules. The other sources
available currently are:

- Synthetic Astaxanthin
- Astaxanthin from Phaffia rhodozyma yeast
- Natural Astaxanthin from food sources, primarily salmon

We will look at each of these alternatives in detail to understand why Natural Astaxanthin from microalgae is clearly the superior choice.

Synthetic Astaxanthin

Synthetic Astaxanthin is the most commonly sold form of Astaxanthin in the world today, but you can't buy it as a supplement for human nutrition because to date, it is not approved by any country's health authority as safe for human consumption. However, most countries do allow it to be sold for use in animal feeds. In fact, if you buy salmon that is not clearly labeled as "wild" or "naturally colored," you're probably eating synthetic Astaxanthin. While this isn't going to kill you, it's certainly not the same as eating fresh, wild salmon with plenty of Natural Astaxanthin (and, incidently, much higher levels of Omega-3 fatty acids than the farmed version). We should take a moment to qualify this: There are farmed salmon appearing in supermarkets recently that are grown under much better conditions, and one of these important conditions is the use of non-synthetic Astaxanthin. One of these natural sources can actually be the same outstanding form of Astaxanthin from microalgae that you commonly find in Astaxanthin supplements on the shelves of health food stores. But the other non-synthetic form that is more commonly used due to its lower cost is from mutated Phaffia yeast, which we'll discuss in detail in the next section.

Synthetic Astaxanthin is produced by an intricate and highly involved process from petrochemicals. That's right—oil! The same thing you put into your car engine's crankcase and the same thing that they make plastic out of is used to produce synthetic Astaxanthin, which is fed to fish and other animals to color them. But even in animals, there is a huge difference between health benefits and even pigmentation when using synthetic Astaxanthin versus algae-based formulas.

Some aquaculture companies are beginning to use Natural Astaxanthin instead of synthetic even though it costs more. Aquaculture is a highly competitive industry, so paying more for a feed ingredient is only done when there is a clear reason why it makes economic sense. And there is. Similar to all the research going on with Natural Astaxanthin for human nutrition, researchers and companies are sponsoring feed trials for animals with Natural Astaxanthin. Some of these trials actually compare the differences between the animals fed the synthetic versus Phaffia-derived and Natural Astaxanthin sources. And what they're finding out is that Natural Astaxanthin is superior to synthetic for promoting health in many different animals. They're even finding that, although synthetic Astaxanthin is much more concentrated than natural as a percentage (synthetic products are sold at an average concentration of 8% - 10% Astaxanthin, whereas Natural Astaxanthin for animal use is sold at concentrations of 1.5% - 2%), Natural Astaxanthin can actually pigment some species of fish better than synthetic.

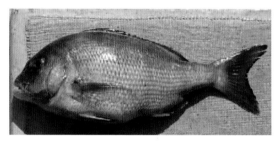

Japanese red sea bream (Pagrus major) pigmented with synthetic Astaxanthin has a dull, sickly color.

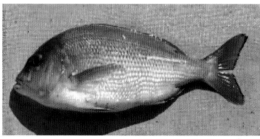

The same species of Japanese red sea bream pigmented with Natural Astaxanthin from Haematococcus microalgae looks healthier and more appetizing. The pigment is more evenly spread throughout the skin of the fish, making it look just like a wild-caught fish.

Photo courtesy of Marubeni Nisshin Feed Co, Japan

One of the main reasons why Natural Astaxanthin works better in pigmenting certain species of fish is because of the fatty acids attached at the ends of the molecule. This esterified version of the Astaxanthin molecule is much better at getting to every part of the body of different animals (and although not clinically proven yet, this is almost undoubtedly true in humans too). Natural Astaxanthin is "systemic"—it gets throughout the body into all the organs, including the skin.

This is why it works so well as an internal sunscreen. This is also why it helps Japanese sea bream fish farmers to have a much better looking end product.

Some of the better tropical fish feed companies are also using Natural Astaxanthin instead of synthetic to help bring out brilliant colors in their customers' fish. By adding a small amount of Natural Astaxanthin into the feed formula, the results can be staggering. Just look at what it can do for the German Peacock fish below:

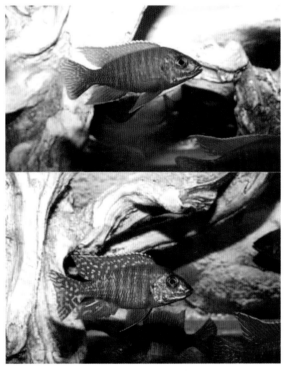

The top fish has no Astaxanthin in the formula, while the bottom fish ate feed with Natural Astaxanthin. The difference in colors and definition is amazing! Just look at how clearly defined the spots are on the bottom fish.

Another important difference is the shape of the synthetic Astaxanthin molecule. Although Natural Astaxanthin, synthetic and Phaffia-derived Astaxanthin all share the same chemical formula, they are all shaped differently. The molecules are different from each other, with the Natural Astaxanthin from microalgae being shaped exactly like the Astaxanthin found in the natural food chain. Synthetic and Phaffia-derived Astaxanthin cannot even be considered the same product as Natural Astaxanthin.

But the most important difference between Natural Astaxanthin and synthetic is how they work. As we examined earlier, Natural Astaxanthin is over 20 times stronger as an antioxidant than synthetic! We also saw instances in animal trials where Natural Astaxanthin helped different species to have higher survival rates, better immunity, fertility and reproduction, and even helped them grow faster. There is no doubt that Natural Astaxanthin is completely different and far superior to synthetic Astaxanthin.

Phaffia Derived Astaxanthin

Phaffia rhodozyma is a yeast that produces Astaxanthin. The problem is, it is not possible to cost effectively produce Astaxanthin using wild strains of Phaffia because they produce no more than 300 ppm of Astaxanthin. Commercial Phaffia used in salmon and trout feeds are mutated strains of Phaffia that produce about 20 times more Astaxanthin than the wild type. The mutation is done using UV light, gamma radiation, or mutagenic chemicals. The mutation process also produces substantial changes in various metabolic pathways (many of them not exclusively related to the production of Astaxanthin) to yield the necessary increment in Astaxanthin production. Thus, Phaffia yeast-derived Astaxanthin has been subjected to considerable genetic manipulation and is not a natural product.

The chemical structure of Astaxanthin from Phaffia is completely different from that of Natural Astaxanthin found in the food chain. Astaxanthin that is ingested by marine animals is always esterified (has one or more fatty acid molecules attached to it), just like Natural Astaxanthin from Haematococcus microalgae. Astaxanthin from Phaffia is non-esterified. It is 100% "free" Astaxanthin, the same type of Astaxanthin that makes up only 5% of the Natural Astaxanthin complex from microalgae. Furthermore, as discussed in the last section, it actually has a different chemical structure than Natural Astaxanthin, and is much more similar to synthetic than it is to Natural Astaxanthin. The difference in structure is in the shape of the molecule. While Natural Astaxanthin from Haematococcus microalgae is practically a carbon copy of the Astaxanthin found in krill, the tiny shrimp that larger marine animals feed on in nature's food chain, Phaffia-derived and synthetic Astaxanthin do not share this shape. When you get right down to it, Phaffia-derived and synthetic Astaxanthin, when compared to Natural Astaxanthin, are two completely different things. And the great additional advantage that Natural Astaxanthin from microalgae has over Phaffia and synthetic is that it comes in a natural, synergistic complex. The complex includes three different types of Astaxanthin, 70% that is monoesterified (with a fatty acid molecule attached to one end), 10% that is diesterified (with fatty acid molecules attached to both ends), and 5% that is the free astaxanthin found predominantly in the Phaffia and synthetic varieties. The remaining 15% is a wonderful blend of supporting carotenoids that make this a truly natural, synergistic product: 6% beta carotene, 5% canthaxanthin and 4% lutein.

Although, unlike synthetic Astaxanthin, Phaffia-derived Astaxanthin is permitted to be sold as a human nutrition supplement in the USA, it is still an inferior form for human consumption and is permitted only with restrictions. Many other countries do not permit this mutated variety. The US FDA, in a letter dated July 17, 2000, allowed the manufacturer of Phaffia-derived Astaxanthin to market the product in the United States with these restrictions:

- Maximum dosage of 2 mg per day
- Only permitted for limited durations of time
- Not permitted for use by children

The restrictions show some serious safety concerns for this mutated yeast product. None of these restrictions apply to Natural Astaxanthin from Haematococcus microalgae, with its extensive safety profile and ten years of public consumption as a supplement.

Natural Astaxanthin from Salmon

If you eat farm raised salmon, which comprises a large majority of the salmon marketed around the world, there is a high probability you're eating synthetic Astaxanthin. There is a chance that you're eating Phaffia, and a very small chance that you're eating Natural Astaxanthin from Haematococcus. Such is the current state of farmed salmon worldwide: Synthetic Astaxanthin dominates the market, Phaffia is a distant second with a small niche, and Natural Astaxanthin from microalgae or krill together hold far less than 1% of the market. And unfortunately, other fish and seafood may also be colored with synthetic Astaxanthin or other unnatural pigments.

Wild salmon is a healthy alternative that contains Natural Astaxanthin, but it can be very hard to find. In fact, even if you think you've bought wild salmon, there's a chance that you're being cheated. Both the New York Times in 2005 and Consumer Reports Magazine in 2006 found widespread cheating—salmon sold as "wild" at much higher prices that was actually farm-raised and synthetically pigmented. And not only are consumers being cheated out of the best Astaxanthin, but farm raised salmon has lower levels of beneficial omega-3 fatty acids as well.

But even if you are successful in finding wild salmon to buy, there are other problems with wild salmon: It is very expensive and may contain high levels of mercury or other unwanted toxins. Because of these problems, the easiest, safest and most cost effective way to get the health benefits of Astaxanthin is to take a high quality Natural Astaxanthin supplement from a respected manufacturer.

Unique Measurement Challenges

As mentioned earlier, Natural Astaxanthin derived from Haematococcus is offered by a few different microalgae farmers. These companies offer a variety of extracted oleoresin (oil-based) Astaxanthin products and Astaxanthin powders for tableting. Unfortunately, the analysis methods for Astaxanthin and the reporting of the Astaxanthin content are not standardized. This can lead to confusion in the marketplace and to consumer products with dosages under that of label claims.

There are two general methods for analyzing the Astaxanthin content of a product: Spectrophotometric analysis and High Pressure Liquid Chromatography (HPLC) analysis. The problem with the spectrophotometric assay method is that, in addition to Astaxanthin, other carotenoids such as lutein, canthaxanthin, and beta carotene are falsely included as Astaxanthin in the results. Of even greater concern, chlorophyll and degradation products of Astaxanthin without health benefits (such as astacene) will also be falsely included as Astaxanthin. Astaxanthin concentrations determined by spectrophotometric analyses can be overstated by 20% - 30%. (The results will definitely be overstated by a minimum of 18%). Some manufacturers try to minimize this overstatement by reporting spectrophotometric analyses results as "Astaxanthin Complex" to indicate that the analysis includes other carotenoids. While this is technically more correct, it does not provide the true level of Astaxanthin in a product, nor does it account for the possible presence of chlorophyll or degradation products of Astaxanthin. Purchasing Astaxanthin from a supplier that uses spectrophotometric analysis means that you can't be sure if your Astaxanthin is really Astaxanthin—it will definitely have other carotenoids and it may very well have chlorophyll and astacene as well that is counted as Astaxanthin!

The most technically sound and accurate method for determining the Astaxanthin content of a product is by HPLC analysis. Determination of the

Astaxanthin content of Haematococcus algae by Cyanotech Corporation's HPLC analytical method has been accepted by the US Food and Drug Administration (21 CFR 73.185), the Canadian Food Inspection Agency (Registration Number 990535) and is used by Japan's official analysis agency, the Japan Food Research Laboratory (JFRL). Cyanotech is widely regarded as the world expert in measuring the esterified Astaxanthin present in Natural Astaxanthin; as a matter of fact, in 2001 a scientist from Cyanotech was invited to Japan to teach the scientists at the Japan Food Research Laboratory how to properly measure esterified Astaxanthin. It is not an easy thing to do.

Below is an HPLC chromatograph showing the carotenoid fraction of Haematococcus microalgae.

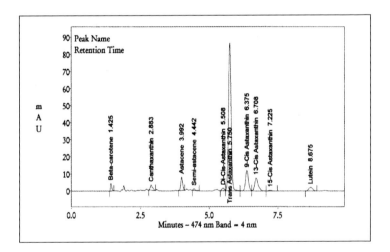

Scientists can read the peaks in this chart to measure the levels of Astaxanthin present in capsules, tablets, or Astaxanthin raw materials. Although much more complicated and requiring further steps, scientists can also use this system to measure Astaxanthin content in foods, animal feeds and cosmetic products. You'll notice that there are small peaks for both astacene and semi-astacene in the chart above. This is normal and pretty much inevitable—some of the Astaxanthin in any product or raw material will have oxidized during handling and broken down into these inert bi-products. One of the biggest problems with the spectrophotometric analysis employed by some Natural Astaxanthin producers is that these useless compounds will be included in the measurement of Astaxanthin for which the company and later, the consumer will be paying. Basically, they're being cheated. And to make matters worse, if the algae are harvested just a little early, there will be another peak on this chart for chlorophyll. Using the spectrophotometric analysis, even the chlorophyll will be counted as Astaxanthin and the consumer will be cheated even more.

To summarize, there is only one proper way to measure Astaxanthin content—HPLC, and the method to measure by this analytical method is very difficult to properly follow. So it's "buyer beware" until the industry can formally standardize a common procedure for measuring Astaxanthin and properly follow it.

CHAPTER 10

Testimonials

> **Publisher's Note:** The testimonials in this book are not intended to imply that Natural Astaxanthin can cure or prevent any disease, nor are they intended as an aid in diagnosing or treating any disease. Also, please note that BioAstin®, AstaZan® and astaXantip® are three different brand names for Natural Astaxanthin and registered trademarks of Cyanotech Corporation, Kailua-Kona, Hawaii, Lifestream International Ltd, Auckland, New Zealand and Asta4you, Gistrup, Denmark respectively.

People taking Astaxanthin report many benefits including increases in stamina and energy. They feel greater strength and recover faster from exercise. They say their skin has better resistance to the sun and improved appearance. They report better immunity and increased resistance to colds and flu. Many also report that Natural Astaxanthin gives them great relief from countless different painful conditions caused by inflammation as well as several other health benefits. Medical doctors and chiropractors swear by it; professional athletes and weekend warriors extol its benefits. Here are some of the many letters that were sent to the offices of Cyanotech in Hawaii, producers of BioAstin® Natural Astaxanthin. While these are not scientific studies, they do show how people feel a difference in their health when using Natural Astaxanthin.

Testimonials from the United States

Medical Doctor says Natural Astaxanthin 'Changed his Life'

I was born and raised in Honolulu. Both of my parents were physicians with me being the fifth generation of physicians on my mother's side. I have been practicing anesthesiology in Honolulu for over twenty-five years. I have spent most of my youth, and as many free hours of my life as possible, in and on the ocean. Unfortunately I have always been exquisitely sensitive to sun exposure, becoming physically ill after a day in the sun, and always getting a burn no matter how much sunscreen, hats, and long shirts I put on. It definitely affected my quality of life, and I started avoiding going outdoors to the detriment of my ingrained psyche that craved being in the sun.

BioAstin [Natural Astaxanthin] literally changed my life, I am outdoors in the sun whenever and for as long as I like. For myself, the increased sun tolerance has been quite remarkable. Most of my surfing and diving friends now use the product.

In my specialty of cardiothoracic anesthesia for open heart surgery and transplantation, the use of pharmacologic doses of free radical scavengers is crucial to survival of the patients whose organ systems are being challenged by the stresses of complex operations. The anesthesia research literature is heavily published in this area. For this reason I have intimate knowledge of how this product BioAstin works, and the potential significance of application in the medical field.

Coincidentally, within a few weeks after I starting taking Astaxanthin, I noticed that it was so much easier to jump out of bed in the morning. The usual stiffness and occasional soreness that would take 15 to 30 minutes to resolve was gone. I didn't think about it much at the time, but looking back at it now, I realize that my physical body regained the smooth, painless functions that I enjoyed in my thirties, almost twenty years ago.

Lastly, some of the older surgeons I work with who have confided in me their own 'aches and pains' have tried BioAstin themselves and been so amazed that they are now recommending it to their patients. (Dr. Robert K. Childs MD, Honolulu, Hawaii)

Professional Triathlete

My name is Tim Marr and I am a professional triathlete from Honolulu, Hawaii. I first discovered BioAstin about 4 years ago, which was when I first started racing triathlons. Racing triathlons in Hawaii involves two things: Heavy exercise and long term sun exposure. With these issues in mind I was looking for a product that would help my performance in those two areas. My solution was BioAstin. Once I started using BioAstin I noticed a significant improvement in overuse injuries as well as long term sun exposure. Antioxidants are the secret to training performance and recovery and BioAstin is packed full of high quality antioxidants. The value of a BioAstin bottle with 60 capsules is a great deal, even as a college student I knew the benefit was well worth the investment. I will be using BioAstin for many years to come, and it will be one of my favorite tools as a professional athlete. I want to thank BioAstin for helping me achieve my goals—it's an important part of all of my results. (Tim Marr, Honolulu, Hawaii. Winner of the 2006 Pan American Long Distance Triathlon — which included a new swim course record — as well as many other races.)

America's Top Freediver— Immunity/Recovery/Less Fatigue

My sport is physically demanding and I train in very extreme conditions. I found out about BioAstin in 2003 and started taking it religiously. I took it on the premise that it would take care of the free radicals in my system which bind to the oxygen molecules and would hinder oxygen uptake. Once I started taking BioAstin I noticed an overall change in my health. I was getting sick far less than previous years. Colds and flu, which are a potential problem for freediving during training and for competition as I push my body to its limits, had become a non-issue for me. On top of this I was noticing changes in my training itself. During dives I found that on my ascent I was getting far less fatigued and absolutely no lactic acid build up in my quadriceps. I was also recovering from the dives much quicker on the surface, which means that I am able to catch my breath far quicker than before. In recent weeks I have conducted my own personal experiment and stopped using BioAstin to see what effects this would have on my body in training. During training dives to 200 feet I was experiencing much fatigue in my quadriceps on my ascent. I was also taking much longer to recover from the dives on the surface than while taking BioAstin. This re-enforced my belief that BioAstin really was making a difference in my diving performances.

Based on my experience with your product I feel very confident and enthusiastic to promote its benefits in regards to the sport of freediving in my National and International appearances at competitions. (Deron Verbeck, America's Top Ranked Freediver, Kailua-Kona, Hawaii)

70 Year Old—Joint Pain/Stamina/Macular Degeneration

My wife and I have been taking BioAstin for almost two years. Our joint pain has gone away or was significantly reduced, in the case of my wife. I work out at a local gym for 2 hours, 6 days a week, riding the bike for 45 - 60 minutes at a time, the rest of the time on strength exercises. I no longer have pain in my knees and my stamina has improved. In addition, I developed a vision problem nine months ago in my right eye which has recently been diagnosed as potentially macular degeneration. I'm not sure this is correct as my vision has been improving each month and my vision has returned almost to what it was prior to the problem occurring. I don't know if BioAstin has anything to do with this but with all the other improvements in my general health it could be the BioAstin along with the exercise. My wife and I will be 70 years old next year and want to continue our good health. (Richard C. Walmer, Fort Myers, Florida)

Reduced Amount of Anti-Inflammatory Medication

I have been taking BioAstin since our anniversary trip to Hawaii in July. In that time I have been able to substantially reduce the amount of anti-inflammatory medication I take for arthritis. Thanks for the great product. (Bob Scharnowske, Alexandria, Indiana)

College Athlete—Sore Hands

I was a collegiate athlete and have had a lot of problems with joint pain in my hands for years. In fact, it gets so bad that I'm unable to hold a newspaper for longer then 5 minutes without my hands and fingers getting sore. I started taking BioAstin about 5 years ago and since taking BioAstin my hands and fingers are 90% better. I started seeing results after the first 2 months. I have tried several different competitive products and within 2 weeks my hands were just as bad as prior to taking BioAstin. I will definitely never use anything else! I'm glad I finally found something that works. (Mark Vieceli, Business Development Manager, Capsugel, a Division of Pfizer, Greenwood, South Carolina)

Energy and Stamina

I first was introduced to BioAstin when we visited Hawaii this last summer. I feel that I have more energy and stamina since I have taken it as a supplement, and include it with my vitamins each day. (Chris Ohrmund, Walnut, California)

113

Immunity/Skin Tone/Exercise Recovery

I am a marathoner and have been taking your product since March 2002. I took one gel before exercise for the first 2 years in accordance with your instructions. Taking the BioAstin made a huge difference in my recovery time as well as allowing me to run pain free on my daily training runs of 6 miles. On my weekend long run of 12 to 18 miles, I do experience a bit of soreness in the calves, and on completing the last Honolulu Marathon 2005, only a bit sore for a day or so. Prior to taking BioAstin, I could expect to be sore for 4 – 5 days. The past year or so I have increased my dosage to 3 per day for short runs and 5 per day for long runs of 12-18 miles.

My immunity is very high as a result of taking BioAstin, I am sick-free year round except for right after the marathon, I am prone to catching the flu or colds. My skin tone is great also.

I am a good spokesman for BioAstin, having many family and friends hooked on your product to whom I send BioAstin as far as Paris, Orlando and California. Keep up the good work. (Dien Truong, Chief Engineer, John A. Burns School of Medicine, Honolulu, Hawaii)

Gum Disease/Tendonitis

I just wanted to let you know about my experience with your BioAstin Astaxanthin supplement. Your company might find this to be very interesting since my benefit was not something I was expecting, namely healing my gum disease. I think the name for gum disease is gingivitis. Anyway, here is my experience.

I began using BioAstin to help with tendonitis in my wrists and forearms and it did really help with that. Prior to my introduction to BioAstin, I had been dealing with regular problems with bleeding and receding gums. I had even resorted to having gum surgery on one particularly bad area. My dentist and hygienist urged me to brush and floss more often than once a day. Despite good intentions, I have never managed to improve my brushing and flossing even to this day. After beginning BioAstin supplementation, my gums began to improve. The hygienist began to find fewer problem areas and pockets each time I had my teeth cleaned. Within a year, I had virtually no gum problems. I was unable to change my brushing and flossing habits and I did not really change my diet or regular supplements during this period. I feel that this dramatic improvement in my gum health can only be attributed to using BioAstin. My dose was two gelcaps per day.

Thanks for your work in developing this wonderful product. (Anton Granger, Captain Cook, Hawaii)

Sunscreen/Joint Pain

My wife and I recently completed a 9,940 mile trip by motorcycle from California, USA to Quebec, Canada and back. We headed east from California through Nevada and Utah in May, 2005 and the temperatures reached over 100 degrees Fahrenheit. We started using BioAstin one week prior to departure and used no sun block for the next 60 days of our ride. I was driving the motorcycle and never had sunburn. My wife Jeanette was behind me and did have sunburn one day in Colorado on her neck, however it tanned and did not peel.

I also usually use glucosamine and chondroitin for joint pain and found I didn't need it when using the BioAstin. This allowed us to carry 1/3 the number of pills we normally carry on such trips. Thanks for a great product. (Russ Taylor, Cayucos, California.)

Pain and Mobility/Healing from Injuries

I first purchased BioAstin in July of 2005. I had problems with my right knee for years, in part due to a pronation problem with my right foot. I finally got custom orthotics, which fixed that problem. However, six months after getting the orthotics, my right knee still hurt.

It hurt getting up or down, and stairs were agony. I couldn't even stretch my leg out straight when lying in bed, it always had to be bent. Nothing I did—rest, exercise, painkillers—helped it heal.

Once I received the BioAstin, I took 3 gelcaps a day. Within 3 weeks, the pain in my right knee was gone for the first time in years. I've continued to take it daily. I have gotten minor injuries in that knee since, and the BioAstin helps the knee heal very quickly. Thank you for giving me real mobility back! (Barbara J. Pfeiffer, Portland, Oregon)

Rheumatoid Arthritis

We started taking BioAstin in June of 2001 while we were visiting the Big Island [Hawaii] for a month. I have had Rheumatoid Arthritis for about 30 years. I first starting having problems when I was in my early 30s. My joints in my fingers were usually very sore and swollen. My feet hurt most of the time when I walked. Over the years I have taken a lot of different medicines, and have found some that have provided much relief from the normal aches and pains, but after I started taking BioAstin, I noticed some of my greatest changes. About a week after I started taking it, I noticed that when we got out of the car after a long day driving, I was not stiff or sore when I stood up. Over the next few months, my hands had less swelling, and were not sore at all. I was able to walk further and enjoy the exercise more because I was not stiff or sore afterwards.

Both my wife and I take BioAstin every day. We walk, on average 6 - 7 miles per day, some days going as far as 8 - 9 miles. We are also both avid bicyclists during the warm months. We have more energy than most friends our age, and have been enjoying excellent physical checkups every year. We look forward to many years of using this product. (Ronald W. Holt, Admin. Officer Emeritus, Medical School Academic Affairs, Madison, Wisconsin)

Bronchitis/Chronic Pain in Tendons/Bleeding Gums

I used BioAstin for one month for the purpose of boosting my immune system because of a stubborn case of bronchitis. The bronchitis, which had been troubling me for four months, disappeared. What I didn't expect was the drastic improvement in inflamed tendons and connective tissue in my shoulder and left knee. Chronic pain in those areas disappeared by the second week of BioAstin usage, along with bleeding of the gums due to a mild case of gingivitis. This is a wonderful product. (Brenda Meechum, Boston, Massachusetts)

Sunscreen/Recovery from Exercise

I began taking BioAstin last spring after reading about it on the Truth Publishing web site. It interested me as I am an 65 year old avid cyclist, so I spend several hours a week in the sun. I don't like to use sunscreen because of the ingredients in it that are considered unsafe by several alternative health sites that I read and trust. I do use extra virgin coconut oil on my skin, but wanted extra protection from a good antioxidant. I used no commercial sunscreen all spring, summer, and fall—had no sunburns even staying out in the sun on my bicycle for 5- 6 hours, 3 or more days a week. I did a total of 3700 miles for the year. The compliment I heard all summer was 'you have a beautiful color tan.' It was glowing and a prettier hue than any other year!

The other reason I chose BioAstin was to help in the recovery time of all that cycling. I was not really that tired and very rarely sore from doing 30 miles or more several times a week. I even did a week long, 341 mile cycling vacation along Lake Michigan with no problems. I will definitely not quit taking this great supplement. (Joann Curtis, Chesterfield, Missouri)

Aching Hands

I have used BioAstin for the last few years and my hands thank you for the comfort I've experienced through consistent use of BioAstin. After about age 40 I started to feel what I can only describe as an aching in my hands and within just weeks of taking BioAstin on a daily basis the ache subsided and hasn't returned since. I also started to put one BioAstin gelcap out for my wife each morning and the crick in her neck from a car accident years ago improved noticeably within just weeks of starting the one-a-day BioAstin regimen. Plain & simple— BioAstin works wonders and I hope to never go without it. (Frank Hart, Poolesville, Maryland)

Bladder Tumors

I have been taking BioAstin for years to keep bladder tumors away. I have not had any more tumors since taking BioAstin. I started taking it when my wife read an article in Women's World Magazine that said that BioAstin was great for preventing tumors, especially bladder tumors. (Robert March, Salt Lake City, Utah)

Cholesterol/Bronchitis

I love BioAstin. My cholesterol dropped from 233 to 180 after taking BioAstin for six months, and I never got the winter bronchitis that I normally get. (Lisa Marie Duncan, Grand Ledge, Michigan)

Knee Problems after Surgery

I'm just writing to tell you about BioAstin, a nutritional supplement I've been taking that really has helped the health of my joints over the past few months. After having surgery on one knee and problems with the other a few years ago, I had recurring problems with my knees. Since I began taking BioAstin, I haven't had any joint pain, despite my history of chronic knee problems. BioAstin also has a very high level of antioxidants, which is important for people like me who live in heavily polluted cities. (Roger Forsberg, Los Angeles, California)

Colds and Flu/Cold Sores

I have used BioAstin for the past few years. Since taking BioAstin, I feel at least I am doing something to combat the negative aspects of free radicals etc., which we are all being bombarded with. I have noticed a distinct decrease in colds and flu, and having previously had the occasional cold sore, I cannot remember when the last one was. Excellent result! (Arlene Meyers, Seattle, WA)

Pre-Cancerous Skin Condition/Pimples/Hair and Nails

A friend that lives in Hawaii first told me about your product about four years ago. He had used it for a while and his pre-cancerous skin condition had cleared up. He is a red-headed carpenter working there in the sun. I have similar skin and I became sun burned often and easily. Since I began taking BioAstin I haven't had one sunburn. The monthly outbreak of pimples I often had has not occurred either. My hair, which has been about the same length for decades grew longer. My fingernails also grew thicker and stronger. I have been so happy with these results that I will continue to take BioAstin and often recommend it to others. (Deborah Dixon, Amesville, Ohio)

Migraines/Improved Health

My husband and I attribute our improved health to BioAstin. For years, I suffered from migraine headaches attributed to food allergies such as wheat and chocolate which are difficult to avoid. Instead of two to three days of painful and building migraines, I can now go for most of each month prior to having a migraine and in fact, with my fingers crossed, I don't recall having one this month (Dec. 2005).

My husband and I were in route to Kauai, Hawaii two summers ago, when he read an article about BioAstin. We spent part of our vacation looking for your product which we found in one of the health food stores. Your product along with trying to apply other healthy lifestyle habits such as exercise have dramatically improved our lives.

Thank you, thank you, thank you. (Dana and Rob Gourley, Sarasota, Florida)

Hawaii's Top Marathon Runner

I used to take various supplements that included antioxidants, Vitamin E & Vitamin C. I also took glucosamine to help joint pain. I started taking BioAstin several years ago and found that it gave me more energy day to day. BioAstin is a very healthy supplement. I have since recommended it to my parents and they too have been taking it daily.

Marathon training is very demanding and BioAstin has helped me recover from intense workouts quicker even though I was getting older. I also found that I no longer needed to take various antioxidants or glucosamine as BioAstin seemed to have benefits of these supplements too. Now I just take BioAstin and Hawaiian Spirulina. (Jonathan Lyau, Hawaii's top finisher in the Honolulu Marathon six straight years, Honolulu, Hawaii)

Competitive Swimmer—Severe Tendonitis

I was a competitive swimmer from the age of 3 through 18, then continued on a limited basis until age 24. After all these years of very heavy training which included 4 hours daily of pool workouts and weight training, working as a lifeguard, competing in rough water swims, training in Junior Lifeguards, and surfing for fun – I developed severe tendonitis in both shoulders and both knees.

My tendonitis starting flaring up when I was 14 years old; it got so bad within that same year I dropped from being number 10 in the nation in sprint events to not even being on the top 50 list. I slept with ice packs on my shoulders and missed a lot of swim workouts. It was difficult to stand up from a crouching position, as the tendonitis in my knees was very painful; walking was painful too. Tendonitis is the reason why I passed up scholarships for college and ultimately stopped competing.

I began taking BioAstin in May 2002, age 29. I started with 1, then 2 BioAstin daily. It took about 4 months for my tendonitis to heal to the point that I did not have pain or notice that it was ever there. Now it is November 2004, I'm still taking 2 BioAstin daily, and still no pain in my shoulders or knees. I have not altered any of my daily routines, diet, or exercise.

I directly attribute my use of BioAstin to the healing of my tendonitis. I had this condition for 15 years, and nothing I did, didn't do, or tried ever worked. I wish this product was around when I was 14 years old, but I'm happy that I have it now. (Nicholle Davis, Kailua-Kona, Hawaii)

Miracle Product/Arthritic Shoulder

This product called 'BioAstin' is nothing short of a miracle! And those of you who know me, realize that I am a person who digs deep to discover the truth of claims like these.

I have been troubled for years with a bad shoulder socket. I could not move my left arm to even wave, and trying to hold my baby grandson was extremely painful, and forget trying to sleep on my left side! My family doctor told me that it was arthritis, and that it came with age...to learn to live with it! I did just that, until on a vacation in Kailua-Kona, Hawaii, I found BioAstin in my hotel gift shop. I had nothing to lose by trying, and after taking a full bottle of this, I had begun to regain the use of my left arm! I had done absolutely nothing differently, in the interim...so I bought another bottle and by the time I had finished that one I had absolutely NO pain in my shoulder or my arm!

What else can I say? It worked wonders for me. (Teresa Windmiller, Grove City, Ohio)

Tendonitis/Bleeding Gums/Sinus Inflammation/Lung Infection

I suffered from joint and tendon inflammation in my left knee, as well as tendonitis in a shoulder. I had started BioAstin for immune system enhancement for a stubborn lung infection. The infection subsided after a few weeks of treatment with BioAstin, and I was surprised to find that the joint and tendon symptoms had also abated. Other symptoms that improved included gum bleeding and sinus inflammation. This product can truly improve general health and a host of specific conditions. (Victor Hamilton, Silva, North Carolina)

Acne/Energy

I originally purchased BioAstin about six weeks ago. My 17 year old son and I began taking it. A few weeks later I noticed an energy increase, and my 17 year old son's (who has had severe acne for about 4 years) face started to clear up. We've used an acne doctor for about 2 ½ years, with only a little success and some side effects from the antibiotics. Never before has his face looked clearer.

You people are on to something, and I just thought I'd say thank you. (Douglas Shaffer, Ortonville, Michigan)

Cancer

I am so encouraged about your product that I just had to write you. I am 56 years old and recovering from chemotherapy and radiation treatments due to breast cancer. They told me it was aggressive, stage III type cancer. During treatment, I have been taking a multi-vitamin, beta glucan, IP-6 and Wobenzym to help my body get stronger.

My last 3 cancer tests during and after chemo were 28, 18 and then 27. Then I started taking BioAstin. Three months later my doctor called me regarding my newest cancer tracer blood test. She told me that the test result was a 15! I told her I thought she made a mistake, and to please check my test results again. She said the 15 was correct! Wow! You can't argue with blood test results.

This is so exciting to me! Thank you for BioAstin! (Marlene Ball, San Pedro, California)

Parkinson's/Creaky Joints

I was diagnosed to have Parkinson's disease in February 2000. For the last six years, I've noticed that I get very sore and creaky in my muscles and joints whenever I finished working in the yard. Sometimes I would have to take a break for a couple of weeks because I became so tired.

Three weeks after taking BioAstin, I found myself able to work 4 hour days in the yard and three times per week on lifting weights without feeling sore...no more creaky joints & limbs or sore muscles anymore. At first I was skeptical about your product, but now I have my wife taking it. As far as my

121

Parkinson's goes, I find that I'm not shaking as much, but perhaps this is from not feeling so sore and exhausted anymore. (Jerry Miki, Kailua-Kona, Hawaii)

Back Pain/Sunburn/Carpal Tunnel Syndrome

I've been using BioAstin Natural Astaxanthin since we heard about it from Mike Adam's health website http://www.newstarget.com and it's amazingly good. It's one of the best antioxidants around and I take two every day and find that my lower back pain after a year now is practically non-existent except on really damp days. I actually stopped taking glucosamine to make sure that it was the Astaxanthin that was doing the good job and it was! Because after I stopped the glucosamine and kept taking the Astaxanthin, my pain didn't come back! And when I went to the Dominican Republic in the blazing 90 degree sun, I didn't get sunburned (and I used only minimum sunscreen once or twice during the day) so that claim is true too! I used to take B6 sometimes when I felt my wrists were acting up from sitting at the keyboard all day, but I don't take B6 because the other claim about alleviating carpel tunnel problems is accurate too. (Patri Ginas, Stormville, New York)

Allergies/Fever Blisters/Knee Pain

I began taking BioAstin several years ago because of severe pain in my knees. At the time, I was also having problems with fever blisters, which had lasted several months. The doctors said my knees had to be operated on, and meanwhile the medicine the doctor was giving me for the fever blisters was only marginally helpful. I was in a great deal of pain with my knees, and the fever blisters were driving me up the wall. The latter did not respond to the old standbys, Camphor-Phenique and Blistex which used to be startlingly effective and now did nothing, and the fever blisters were lasting much longer than is normally expected.

Within a week of taking BioAstin, one per day, I noticed the fever blisters clearing up. Likewise, the pain in my knees went away. In addition, I discovered that within a few hours of taking the BioAstin, my eyes were much better; this was a daily event, it did not seem to last for long, but was dramatic.

A few months ago I realized that within a few hours after taking BioAstin, my allergies cleared up. I started taking the BioAstin three times a day, and stopped having to take prescription medicines.

To sum up, taking BioAstin has reduced my allergies, my knee pain, and my fever blister problem to a point where they are no longer major disruptions in my life, and without taking medications which would cost hundreds of dollars and might have side effects. And it's saving me the time and expense of knee surgery. (Ron Kelley, Fish Camp, California)

Tendonitis/Periodontal Disease

I am writing this letter to express my sincere appreciation for BioAstin. I have never before written a company a testimonial, but I feel compelled to for this wonderful product. I want to share my story of unexpected healing with you.

A wise friend recommended I try two gel caps of BioAstin to help alleviate pain I was experiencing due to tendonitis in my wrists and elbows. Remarkably, the irritating pain gradually subsided within two months of taking the Astaxanthin supplement. I am thankful for this relief, however, I believe BioAstin had another surprisingly wonderful effect on my body.

For years, I had been struggling with periodontal disease. Although I tried to increase flossing and brushing, my dentist said my gums were receding and I should consider surgery. After a year of supplementing my regular diet with BioAstin and not changing my flossing and brushing routine, my gums improved dramatically. The only variable was BioAstin and therefore, I think that the Astaxanthin supplement is responsible for my spectacular recovery. (Will Jacobson, South Kona, Hawaii)

Joint Pain—Better Results than Glucosamine & Sam-E

I was taking Sam-E, chondroitin sulfate, and glucosamine for joint pain due to old injuries to wrist and knees for years with reasonable results. A good friend told me that he simply took your BioAstin product for those same symptoms with excellent results. I had previously used BioAstin for eye care and resistance to ultraviolet rays from lots of sun exposure. So now I have eliminated the other joint stuff for several months while trying BioAstin as a substitute. The results have been remarkably good. I appreciate the benefits, and of course the significant savings. Great Job! (Leimana Pelton, founder of Bamboo Village Hawaii, a nonprofit corporation)

123

Arthritis/Skin Condition

My wife and I have been taking BioAstin for about a year for our arthritis and we don't have joint pain any longer. In addition I've had a chronic skin condition with a severe rash for most of my adult life. It's now in remission and in a very calm state. It hasn't been this way in over 25 years and I believe that the BioAstin has something to do with it. In any event I'm not stopping the BioAstin. All my adult family is now taking BioAstin and many of my friends. It's a great product. (Brandon Finberg, New York City)

Testimonials from Around the World

Energy/Exercise Recovery/Sun Protection

When this new product came onto the New Zealand market I read all the research and marveled at the proclaimed health benefits. I tend to be somewhat cynical about health product claims and look for clinical trials and proven efficacy. When it comes to my personal adoption of any health product, I am a challenge to convert, always having to prove and experience first-hand the health benefits for myself; there is certainly no 'placebo effect' with me!

My lifestyle is hectic, as a national sales manager, frequently traveling throughout New Zealand and as a father of a 5 month old baby. My partner and I are fully committed to sporting and cultural participation so our life is always on the go. Prior to taking AstaZan® [Natural Astaxanthin] I had been taking a multivitamin/mineral and fish oil daily. I started taking AstaZan 6 weeks ago. Within the first week I noticed that my energy levels were improving. By the second week I noticed that my recovery from running 45 minutes 5 days a week was clearly evident. My previous sore joints, muscle and tendon tenderness after each run had all but dissipated for the first time in my life.

The other very noticeable benefit is that AstaZan appears to help prevent my skin from burning. With New Zealand's harsh sun with ozone damage I generally tend to burn quite quickly. Having taken AstaZan for 6 weeks I was out gardening in shorts and singlet from 10 AM through till 6:30 PM recently on a very hot sunny day. Normally I would be very badly sunburned being out this long in these conditions, no matter how much I plastered on sunblock. My partner and I were absolutely astonished to learn that I did not get sunburned at all!

124

I attribute this totally to AstaZan.

So if you are looking for more energy, greater recovery after exercise and sun protection I personally recommend Lifestream's AstaZan. It works for me, and remember, I am the world's greatest health cynic! (Chris Ward, Auckland, New Zealand)

Skin Improvement/Wrinkles/Energy

I would like to share good news with you because I have become healthy and can concentrate more on my work lately. This is because I found a perfect product called 'BioAstin.' It is the best healthy vitamin I have ever seen. After I took it for one week, I felt OK, but nothing happened to my body, but I didn't stop—I took it every day. Three weeks later I felt that it was working, and I also felt that I got more energy every day without sleeping or exercising more. I found that by taking BioAstin once a day my wrinkles are getting fewer and disappearing. Nowadays, I get a lot of energy ever day, and my skin gets more shining and more spotless, and my wrinkles are gone! It is an amazing product and I love it so much. Hurry to try it! (Sophie Su Chen, Taipei, Taiwan)

Sun Allergy/Aches & Pains

I first saw the article about BioAstin in the Daily Mail newspaper way back in April of this year. I read about a lady who suffered, as I did, from not only allergy to the sun, but sensitivity to sun lotions and cream. I was dubious about the claims made about BioAstin but willing to try anything once, at least! For the first time in a very long time, I was able to be out in the sun without ending up with an urticaria rash (allergic reaction like nettle rash). I don't sunbathe because of my allergy but even a few minutes walking a few steps in my garden would have been long enough to be badly affected, before taking BioAstin. I believe BioAstin has also reduced my aches and pains. (Lady Joan G. Johnston, Inverness, Scotland)

Chiropractor—Athletic Performance/Lymphatic Drainage

I have used AstaZan for my athletic patients involved in all kinds of various sports to enhance performance as AstaZan increases one's recovery rate, decreasing sore muscles, lactic acid build up and muscle strains that can lead to injury. I'd highly recommend AstaZan to any athlete that wants to reach the peak of their game.

I have also used AstaZan for patients with lymphatic drainage issues. It appears to help ease some of the pain associated with swelling the lymphatic vessels as well as helps to rid the fluid to some extent. In these individuals other supplements were given as well and the cause of fluid build up should always be determined. Patients I have used AstaZan with include cancer patients who have had lymph tissue removed, fluid retentive patients, those that complain of premenstrual breast soreness and those whose ankles swell after periods of standing on one's feet. These are only a few conditions to consider the use of AstaZan with. (Dr. Joy White, Doctor of Chiropractic, Rangiora, New Zealand)

Joint Pain/Sunscreen

I felt that I had to write to you to say how delighted I am with the BioAstin capsules. When I was only 38 years old, unfortunately I had to have a hysterectomy. Because of this I have had to have HRT implants. Since then I have suffered with severe joint pain, which got progressively worse over a period of time. My doctor just said that I would have to learn to live with it as it was most probably due to an early menopause. I tried various supplements that had been recommended to me, but they didn't seem to help at all. Before the operation, I loved being in the sun, but after my hysterectomy, I seemed to go through many changes, my skin being one of them. I found that I would burn in the sun and my skin would become irritated. When I saw BioAstin being featured on the 'This Morning' program, I thought that I would try it. I was delighted with the way it helped to protect me in the sun, but I was more delighted with how it has helped my aching joints. After taking if for a period of time, I noticed a dramatic difference in my joints; I am no longer in pain and also my joints feel more supple. It is wonderful, I no longer feel like an 'old woman.' (Jeanne Higson, Lancaster, England)

Energy

I felt that I had to write to you, to let you know how pleased both my wife and I are with your product BioAstin. We purchased some a little while ago and already we are both feeling the benefits of it. Several years ago, my wife, who incidentally was a hospital nurse for 35 years, developed painful and debilitating arthritis in her left knee, this triggered off a bacterial infection and she became extremely ill. I was very concerned about her, as she was on loads of drugs to combat the effects of her illness. She was so ill that she had to give up nursing which upset her greatly.

Eventually, she was given a knee replacement and although this did help with the pain and helped to clear up the bacterial infection, after years of illness, it left my wife very tired and with very little or no energy. She found it difficult to do most things that required any stamina, she had to have a nap most afternoons and was in bed by 10:00 PM most evenings.

However, after just a short period of taking the maximum dose [12 mg per day] of BioAstin, my wife has visibly more energy. She can do the housework and other tasks with no discomfort, she doesn't need to rest so often and has even planned day trips out, something she could not have even contemplated before. It is wonderful to see her so happy and positive again.

I have also felt the benefits of BioAstin, I have more energy and generally feel better all around. But, most importantly, it is wonderful to see my wife having more energy, as she did before her knee problems.

We are so grateful to you and will be recommending BioAstin to all our friends and family. (Graham Davies, Grendon, North Atherstone, UK)

Arthritis/Repetitive Stress Injury

I would like to give your company a standing ovation for your AstaZan. Not only has it helped incredibly with my Repetitive Stress Injury [Carpal Tunnel Syndrome] but also seems to have given me greater mobility and relatively pain free arthritis. It works and so well. I have more energy and a wonderful feeling of serenity has come over me which I know is beyond the effects of any health product I have ever tried. The only draw back I have experienced is keeping myself with personal stock as I have shared with at least a dozen people who all have experienced the same types of wonderful benefits. If you do testimonials please include mine as I shall be forever grateful and a steady customer. Thank you so much. (Robert Rizic, Inglewood, New Zealand)

Cold Sores

For twenty-five years I have suffered with horrendous cold sores on my lips, particularly when I have been in the sun. Even walking around on holiday to do some shopping, I had to protect myself with children's factor 50 sun cream. Every holiday was marred by these terrible cold sores unless I used a sunblock. Once I had them it ruined my holiday, and it could take weeks to clear up. This was very debilitating. On one occasion when they were at their worst, I was unable to eat properly for three days.

Since April I have been taking a BioAstin capsule every day and have not had any cold sores this summer. I am so relieved to have found something at last that seems to prevent them. It is also wonderful not to burn in the sun any more, which is something that both my husband and I did before taking BioAstin. (Coral Guise-Smith, Alicante, Spain)

Gum Disease/Gingivitis

I was given a recommendation for BioAstin by a friend for treating gum disease. Having used it for only 2 weeks, the progressive gingivitis stopped, and I have no irritation in my gums whatsoever. Fantastic! (Tim Watson, Corsham, Wiltshire, United Kingdom)

Carpal Tunnel Syndrome/Pain from Playing Guitar

Before I started using BioAstin, I suffered a tremendous amount of pain every time I played guitar. I was in so much pain I sold all of my equipment, 3 very expensive guitars, 2 amps and a whole load of effect pedals. I thought I'd never be able to play guitar again as I discovered I had Carpal Tunnel Syndrome. I tried just about everything I knew of; not even my doctor could help, all he could do was mask the pain.

I took twice the stated dose of BioAstin (8 mg per day) and my pain disappeared within days. In fact one week later I could play guitar again! Now I've bought some brand new equipment and I'm playing even better than I used to.

Based on my experience I think BioAstin is brilliant. I would recommend it to anyone that has any kind of pain (like I had) to try this first. I cannot thank you enough. (Clive Cable, Steepleton, Dorchester, England)

Injury Recovery/Recovery from Exercise

In March 2000, I was in a rear end vehicle collision which occurred at a highway speed of 55 mph. I experienced a severe whiplash injury as I was the driver of the rear ended vehicle – severe neck pain on the left side.

I went to physiotherapy over the next four years with some success but my injury always seemed to resurface. After a doctor's visit in the spring of 2004, my doctor gave me a referral for another round of physiotherapy to treat the motor vehicle accident injury. I said to myself that was enough and the search began for an alternative treatment.

Within six months of taking BioAstin, the muscle mass on the left side of my neck was gone. My physiotherapist couldn't believe it. BioAstin has reduced the number of days of recovery after any significant amount of labor or exercise. It doesn't take three days to recover from one day of active living. It has allowed me to move forward in my life and finally put the motor vehicle accident injury behind me. Thank you! (Nancy Yeo, Stratford, Prince Edward Island, Canada)

Eyesight/Clarity of Vision

My wife is a health nut and I'm anything but. So it was with some skepticism and more for her benefit that I started taking Lifestream AstaZan. I am quite badly short sighted (literally and metaphorically as it turns out) but wear glasses that quite adequately correct my vision. After taking one Lifestream AstaZan capsule a day for 10 days I noticed added clarity of vision and the ability to see more detail at longer distances. Any other health benefits Lifestream AstaZan can offer me are just a bonus as far as I'm concerned. (Rohan Marx, Hamilton, New Zealand)

Slipped Disk

A slipped disc in my back turned my life upside down two years ago. The bad pain forced me to be off work for a longer period, with the result that I lost my job. Not until I began to take a dietary supplement containing a strong antioxidant was I able to get so much control of the pain that I now am able to live a fairly good life again.

I will never let go of this dietary supplement astaXantip® [Natural Astaxanthin] again. The remedy is an extract from algae which grows in Hawaii, and is known as a very strong antioxidant.

I got the dietary supplement recommended by a girlfriend who had positive experiences with it herself. In March last year I began to take it. I was willing to try everything because I was so ill from pain at that time. When the pain was at the worst I had to crawl round my home. Some times I took 16 painkillers each day.

Big was my surprise when I felt a distinct recovery after just five days with astaXantip. As it often happens, the first reaction was a worsening before I felt the positive effect. The first couple of days after I took the dietary supplement it felt like I had the flu, and I had to stay in bed for a couple of days.

For the first time in two years I had no pain when I got out of my bed again. I expected the pain to return shortly after, but it has not happened. I have to take two gelcaps a day, one in the morning and one in the late afternoon. I have tried to reduce my dose to 1 gelcap, but the pain turns back within 10-12 hours, so it is not enough.

I have had a side effect from astaXantip, as my menstrual pain, which has plagued me for many years have disappeared. I have also suffered a lot from sinusitis, and apparently the dietary supplement has removed that too. (Anne Mette Madsen, Aabybro, Denmark)

Sunscreen/Energy

I am very pleased with the results I have had with using BioAstin. BioAstin has not only helped to protect me from the sun, I do not burn so badly as before and I seem to be much browner than usual, but I feel so much better generally. I am 65 years old and am a manual worker, so naturally at my age, I find this type of work very tiring some times. But now, I have loads more energy and do not find it quite so difficult, this has made such a big difference to me, especially with my type of work. I do not get so tired now and feel so much better, particularly in the mornings. I think that this is a great product and I will continue to take it all the time. (Mr. A. Keyes, Wimbledon, London, England)

Sunscreen/Soreness after Exercise

Yesterday I was in the sun all day, I moved 7 plants in the garden, then got a trailer load of stones and re-laid the garden, then built a frame and put up a brush stick fence. I was occasionally wearing a shirt but most of the time I was just in shorts and work shoes. I have a little red tinge around my forearms and a tiny tinge on my neck but not even enough so you would notice. I am blown away. I was out for half the time earlier this year with a shirt on and got fried—

burned and sore. This time no burn, no soreness and out in the sun working from 8 AM 'til 9:40 PM and my skin feels amazing. I have been taking AstaZan for 3 weeks at 3 capsules per day and this is clearly what has protected me from the sun. I was sold before on its 'work hard or exercise and feel no pain or soreness the next day' effect but this is a whole other level and shows what an amazing product AstaZan really is. I am genuinely amazed. (Jason Bennett, Auckland, New Zealand)

Stomach Problems/Aching Knees and Joints

I have suffered for many years with my stomach, I have an acid problem and have to take medication. To my dismay some weeks before my holiday, I developed some problems with my stomach. I had a constant feeling of being too full and 'blown out' all the time, and my stomach would swell up after I had eaten. This was extremely uncomfortable and I couldn't even bear to wear any tight fitting clothing. I went to the doctors, but he suggested that I return after my holiday, as he didn't want to give me any medication before my holiday in case it did not agree with me.

I bought some BioAstin after reading about it and thought that I would try some to stop me from sun burning when I went on holiday. I had also read that it can help with stomach problems, so hoped that it would perhaps alleviate my discomfort. To my delight it did, and by the time I had returned from my holiday, I had no discomfort at all and the problem has cleared up completely. I was so pleased not to have to return to the doctors for more medication.

I shall continue to take BioAstin, not only to protect me as an antioxidant, but to help with my aching knees and joints and of course to alleviate my stomach problems. (John O'Grady, Watford, Herts, England)

Vitiligo [Skin Condition]

I first saw an item on the 'Good Morning' television program regarding BioAstin. A lady who was being interviewed stated that she had extremely sensitive skin and also said that she burned very quickly when she was out in the sun. After taking BioAstin, she was very impressed and found that she didn't burn at all. I was so inspired that I decided to give BioAstin a try for myself, as I suffer from Vitiligo. (This is a skin condition which leaves areas of skin without any melanin—a substance which turns your skin brown when you go out in the sun.

131

It is extremely difficult to go out in the sun with this condition because the white patches have no protection and are very sensitive and burn very easily.)

I have found BioAstin to be a superb product and have now been taking it since 2002 and have not burned once! Also, I have had the best tans ever since taking the capsules and will certainly continue to take this wonderful product. BioAstin has certainly changed my life considerably with regard to holidays and when the sun shines! I would recommend BioAstin to anyone who burns or who suffers like myself with Vitiligo. (Stephanie Vail, Brentwood, Essex, UK)

Tennis Elbow and Sunburn

I have been using BioAstin in the UK for 4 years. I initially took it to help prevent sunburn on holiday and found it fantastic. At the time I was also suffering from 'Tennis Elbow' and gave no thought to the fact that BioAstin is good for joints. The improvement in my elbow has been dramatic so instead of taking from May to August to help protect the skin from the sun I now take it all year round as it deals with both conditions at once. (Elizabeth Littler, Kidderminster, Worcestershire, UK)

References

Akyon, Y. (2002). "Effects of antioxidants on the immune response of Helicobacter pylori." Clinical Microbiology and Infection. 8(7):438-41.

Ames, B., Shigenaga, M. (1992). "Oxidants are a major contributor to aging." Ann. N.Y. Acad. Sci. 663:85-96.

Ames, B., Shigenaga, M., Hagen, T. (1993). "Oxidants, antioxidants and the degenerative diseases of aging." Proc. Natl. Acad. Sci. 90(17):7915-7922.

Anderson, M. (2004). "A preliminary investigation of the enzymatic inhibition of 5alpha-reduction and growth of prostatic carcinoma cell line LNCap-FGC by natural astaxanthin and Saw Palmetto lipid extract in vitro." Journal of Herbal Pharmacotherapy. 5(1):17-26.

Anderson, M. (2001). "Method of inhibiting 5alpha-reductase with astaxanthin" United States Patent 6,277,417.

Aoi, W., Naito, Y., Sakuma, K., Kuchide, M., Tokuda, H., Maoka, T., Toyokuni, S., Oka, S., Yasuhara, M., Yoshikawa, T. (2003). "Astaxanthin limits exercise-induced skeletal and cardiac muscle damage in mice." Antioxidants & Redox Signaling. 5(1):139-44.

Aquis, R., Wattanabe, T., Satoh, S., Kiron, V., Imaizumi, H., Yamazaki, T., Kawano, K. (2001). "Supplementation of paprika as a carotenoid source in soft-dry pellets for broodstock yellow-tail." Seriola quinqueradiata (Temminck and Schlegel). Aquaculture Research. 32(1):263-272.

Arakane, K. (2002). "Superior Skin Protection by Astaxanthin." Carotenoid Research. Volume 5, April 2002.

Arakane, K. (2001). "Superior Skin Protection by Astaxanthin." Presentation at the 15th annual meeting on carotenoid research, September 2001, Toyama, Japan.

Bagchi, D. (2001). "Oxygen Free Radical Scavenging Abilities of Vitamins C, E, B-Carotene, Pycnogenol, Grape Seed Proanthocyanidin Extract, Astaxanthin and BioAstin in Vitro." On file at Cyanotech Corporation.

Baskin, C., Hinchcliff, K., DiSilvestro, R., Reinhart, G., Hayek, M., Chew, B., Burr, J., Swenson, R. (2000). "Effects of dietary antioxidant supplementation on oxidative damage and resistance to oxidative damage during prolonged exercise in sled dogs." Am. J. Vet. Res. 61(8):886-891.

Bates, C., van Dam, D., Horrobin, D., Morse, N., Huang, Y., Manku., M. (1985). "Plasma essential fatty acids in pure and mixed race American Indians on and off a diet exceptionally rich in salmon." Prostaglandins Leukot. Med. 17, 77.

Bennedsen, M., Wang, X., Willen, R., Wadstrom, T., Andersen, L. (1999). "Treatment of H. pylori infected mice with antioxidant astaxanthin reduces gastric inflammation, bacterial load and modulates cytokine release by splenocytes." Immunology Letters. 70(3):185-9.

Bertram, J. (1999). "Carotenoids and gene regulation.", Nutr. Rev. 57, 182.

Beutner, S., Bloedorn, B., Frixel, S., Blanco, I., Hoffmann, T., Martin, H., Mayer, B., Noack, P., Ruck, C., Schmidt, M., Schulke, I., Sell, S., Ernst, H., Haremza, S., Seybold, G., Sies, H., Stahl, W., Walsh, R. (2000). "Quantitative assessment of antioxidant properties of natural colorants and phytochemicals: carotenoids, flavonoids, phenols and indigoids. The role of B-carotene in antioxidant functions." Journal of the Science of Food and Agriculture. 81:559-568.

Black, H. (1998). "Radical interception by carotenoids and effects on UV carcinogenesis." Nutrition and Cancer. 31(3):212-7.

Brunswick Laboratories. (2004). In-vitro testing. On file at Cyanotech Corporation.

Carper, J. (2005). "Eat Smart." USA Weekend Magazine. August 7, 2005.

133

Chew, B. Park, J. (2006). US Patent Application #20060217445.

Chew, B., Park, J. (2004). "Carotenoid action on the immune reponse." The Journal of Nutrition. 134(1):257S-261S.

Chew, B., Park, J., Chyun, J., Mahoney, M., Line, L. (2003). "Astaxanthin Stimulates Immune Response in Humans in a Double Blind Study." Presented at the Supply Side West International Trade Show and Conference, October 1-3, 2003.

Chew, B., Wong, M., Park, J., Wong, T. (1999). "Dietary beta-carotene and astaxanthin but not canthaxanthin stimulate splenocyte function in mice." Anticancer Research. 19(6B):5223-7.

Chew, B., Park, J., Wong, M., Wong, T. (1999). "A comparison of the anticancer activities of dietary B-carotene, canthaxanthin and astaxanthin in mice in vivo." Anticancer Research. 19(3A):1849-53.

Christiansen, R., Lie, O., Torrissen, O. (1995). "Growth and survival of Atlantic salmon, Salmo salar L., fed different dietary levels of astaxanthin. First-feeding fry." Aquaculture Nutrition. 1:189-198.

Christiansen, R., Glette, J., Lie, O., Torrissen, O., Waagbo, R. (1995). "Antioxidant status and immunity in Atlantic Salmon; Almo salar L., fed semi-purified diets with and without astaxanthin supplementation." Journal of Fish Disease. 18:317-328.

Clegg, D., Reda, D., Harris, C., Klein, M., O'Dell, J., Hooper, M., Bradley, J., Bingham, C., Weisman, M., Jackson, C., Lane, N., Cush, J., Moreland, L., Schumaker, H., Oddis, C., Wolfe, F., Molitor, J., Yokum, D., Schnitzer, T., Furst, D., Sawitzke, A., Shi, H., Brandt, K., Moskowitz, R., Williams, H. (2006). "Glucosamine, Chondroitin Sulfate and the two in combination for painful knee osteoarthritis." New England Journal of Medicine. 354(8):795-808.

Cole, G. (2005). Professor of Medicine and Neurology at UCLA, as reported to Anne Underwood, Newsweek Magazine, "Special Summer Issue," August 2005. Pg. 26-28.

Comhaire, F., El Garem, Y., Mahmoud, A., Eertmans, F., Schoonjans, F. (2005). "Combined conventional/ antioxidant "Astaxanthin" treatment for male infertility: A double blind randomized trial." Asian J. Andrology. 7(3):257-262.

Comhaire, F., Mahmoud, A. (2003). "The role of food supplements in the treatment of the infertile man." Reproductive BioMedicine Online. 7(4):385-391(7).

Darachai, J., Piyatiratitivorakul, S., Menasveta, P. (1999). "Effect of Astaxanthin on Stress Resistance of Penaeus monodon Larvae." Proceedings of the 37th Kasetsart University Annual Conference, Bangkok, Thailand. Text & Journal Publication Co. Pg. 240-245

Darachai, J., Piyatiratitivorakul, S., Kittakoop, P., Nitithamyong, C., Menasveta, P. (1998). "Effects of Astaxanthin on Larval Growth and Survival of the Giant Tiger Prawn, Penaeus monodon." Advances in shrimp biotechnology. Pg 117-21.

Davies, K. (1995). "Oxidative stress: the paradox of aerobic life." Biochem. Soc. Symp. 61, 1.

Dekkers, J., van Doornen, L., Kemper, H. (1996). "The role of antioxidant vitamins and enzymes in the prevention of exercise-induced muscle damage." Sports Med. 21(3):213-238.

Dore, J. (2003). "Astaxanthin and Cancer Chemoprevention." Published in "Phytopharmaceuticals in Cancer Chemoprevention." Edited by Debassis Bagchi and Harry Preuss. CRC Press. 2005. Pg 555-574.

Dore, J. (2002). "BioAstin Safety Profile." Cyanotech Technical Bulletin Ax-072. On file at Cyanotech Corporation.

Eastwood, M. (1999). "Interaction of dietary antioxidants in vivo: how fruit and vegetables prevent disease?" Q. J. Med. 92, 527.

Esterbauer, H., Gebicki, J., Puhl, H., Jurgens, G. (1992). "The role of lipid peroxidation and antioxidants in oxidative modification of LDL." Free Rad. Biol. Med. 13:341-390.

Fry, A. (2001). "Astaxanthin Clinical Trial for Delayed Onset Muscular Soreness." Human Performance Laboratories. The University of Memphis. Report 1, August 16, 2001.

Fry, A., Schilling, B., Chiu, L., Hori, N., Weiss, L. (2004) "Astaxanthin Supplementation." Human

134

Performance Laboratories. The University of Memphis. Report 2, May 2004.

Garem, Y., Lignell, A., Comhaire, F. (2002). "Natural Astaxanthin Improves Semen Quality in Infertile Men." Unpublished study.

Goldfarb, A. (1999). "Nutritional antioxidants as therapeutic and preventative modalities in exercise-induced muscle damage." Can. J. Appl. Physiol. 24(3):249-266.

Gradelet, S., Le Bon, A., Berges, R., Suschetet, M., Astorg, P. (1998). "Dietary carotenoids inhibit aflatoxin B1-induced liver preneoplastic foci and DNA damage in the rat: role of the modulation of aflatoxin B1 metabolism." Carcinogenesis. 19(3):403-411.

Gradelet, S., Astorg, P., Le Bon, A., Berges, R., Suschetet, M. (1997). "Modulation of aflatoxin B1 carcinogenicity, genotoxicity and metabolism in rat liver by dietary carotenoids: evidence for a protective effect of CYP1A inducers." Cancer Lett. 114(1-2):221-223.

Gross, G., Lockwood, S. (2005). "Acute and chronic administration of disodium disuccinate astaxanthin (Cardax) produces marked cardioprotection in dog hearts." Molecular and cellular biochemistry. 272(1-2):221-7.

Gross, G, Lockwood, S. (2004). "Cardioprotection and myocardial salvage by a disodium disuccinate astaxanthin derivative (Cardax™). Life Sci. 75:215-24.

Guerin, M., Huntley, M., Olaizola, M. (2002). "Haematococcus astaxanthin: health and nutrition applications." Presented at the 1st Congress of the International Society for Applied Phycology/9th International Congress on Applied Phycology, May 26-30, 2002, Almeria, Spain.

Hansen, K., Tauson, A., Inborr, J. (2001). "Effect of supplementation with the antioxidant astaxanthin on reproduction, pre-weaning growth performance of kits and daily milk intake in mink." Journal of reproduction and fertility. 57:331-4.

Harman, D. (1981). "The aging process." Proc. Natl. Acad. Sci. 78:7124-7128.

Holick, C., Michaud, D., Stolzenberg-Soloman, R., Mayne, S., Pietinen, P., Taylor, P., Virtamo, J., Albanes, D. (2002). "Dietary carotenoids, serum beta carotene, and retinol and risk of lung cancer in the Alpha-Tocopherol, Beta Carotene cohort study." Am. J. Epidemiol. 156, 536.

Hussein, G., Nakagawa, T., Goto, H., Shimada, Y., Matsumoto, K., Sankawa, U., Watanabe, H. (2006). "Astaxanthin ameliorates features of metabolic syndrome in SHR/NDmcr-cp." Life Sciences.

Hussein, G., Nakamura, M., Zhao, Q., Iguchi, T., Goto, H., Sankawa, U., Watanabe, H. (2005a). "Antihypertensive and neuroprotective effects of astaxanthin in experimental animals." Biological and Pharmaceutical Bulletin. 28(1):47-52.

Hussein, G., Goto, H., Oda, S., Iguchi, T., Sankawa, U., Matsumoto, K., Watanabe, H. (2005b) "Antihypertensive potential and mechanism of action of astaxanthin: II. Vascular reactivity and hemorheology in spontaneously hypertensive rats." Biological and pharmaceutical bulletin. 28(6):967-71.

Ikeuchi, M., Koyama, T., Takahashi, J., Yazawa, K. (2006). "Effects of astaxanthin supplementation on exercise-induced fatigue in mice." Biological and Pharmaceutical Bulletin. 29(10):2106-10.

Ilyasov, Y., Golovin, P. (2003). "The effect of NatuRose® on growth, survival and physiological state of two-year-old marketable sturgeons." On file at Cyanotech Corporation.

Iwamoto, T., Hosoda, K., Hirano, R., Kurata, H., Matsumoto, A., Miki, W., Kamiyama, M., Itakura, H., Yamamoto, S., Kondo, K. (2000). "Inhibition of low-density lipoprotein oxidation by astaxanthin." Journal of Atherosclerosis Thrombosis. 7(4):216-22.

Jyonouchi, H., Sun, S., Iijima, K., Gross, M. (2000). "Antitumor activity of astaxanthin and its mode of action." Nutrition and Cancer. 36(1):59–65.

Jyonouchi, H., Sun, S., Mizokami, M., Gross, M. (1996). "Effects of various carotenoids on cloned, effector-stage T-helper cell activity." Nutrition and Cancer. 26(3):313-24.

Jyonouchi, H., Sun, S., Gross, M. (1995). "Astaxanthin, a carotenoid without vitamin A activity, augments antibody responses in cultures including T-helper cell clones and suboptimal doses of antigen." J. Nutr. 125(10):2483-2492.

Jyonouchi, H., Sun, S., Gross, M. (1995). "Effect of carotenoids on in vitro immunoglobulin production by human peripheral blood mononuclear cells: astaxanthin, a carotenoid without vitamin A activity, enhances in vitro immunoglobulin production in response to a T-dependent stimulant and antigen." Nutrition and Cancer. 23(2):171-183.

Jyonouchi, H., Zhang, L., Gross, M., Tomita, Y. (1994). "Immunomodulating actions of carotenoids: enhancement of in vivo and in vitro antibody production to T-dependent antigens." Nutrition and Cancer. 21(1):47-58.

Jyonouchi, H., Zhang, L., Tomita, Y. (1993). "Studies of immunomodulating actions of carotenoids. II. Astaxanthin enhances in vitro antibody production to T-dependent antigens without facilitating polyclonal B-cell activation." Nutrition and Cancer. 19(3):269-80.

Jyonouchi, H., Hill, R., Tomita, Y., Good, R. (1991). "Studies of immunomodulating actions of carotenoids. I. Effects of beta-carotene and astaxanthin on murine lymphocyte functions and cell surface marker expression in in-vitro culture system." Nutrition and Cancer. 16(2):93-105.

Kang, J., Kim, S., Kim, H. (2001). "Effect of astaxanthin on the hepatotoxicity, lipid peroxidation and antioxidative enzymes in the liver of CCl4-treated rats." Methods and findings in experimental and clinical pharmacology. 23(2):79-84.

Kim, H., Park, J., Chew, B. (2001). "B-carotene and astaxanthin inhibit mammary tumor cell growth and induce apoptosis in mice in vitro." FASEB J. 15, A298.

Kim, J., Kim, Y., Song, G., Park, J., Chang, H. (2005a). "Protective effect of astaxanthin on naproxen-induced gastric antral ulceration in rats." European Journal of Pharmacology. 514(1):53-9.

Kim, J., Choi, S., Choi, S., Kim, H., Chang, H. (2005b). "Suppressive effect of astaxanthin isolated from the Xanthophyllomyces dendrorhous mutant on ethanol-induced gastric mucosal injury in rats." Bioscience, Biotechnology, and Biochemistry. 69(7):1300-5

Kozuki, Y., Miura, Y., Yagasaki, K. (2000). "Inhibitory effects of carotenoids on the invasion of rat ascites hepatoma cells in culture." Cancer Lett. 151, 111.

Kudo, Y., Nakajima, R., Matsumoto, N. (2002). "Effects of astaxanthin on brain damages due to ischemia" Carotenoid Science. 5,25.

Kurashige, M., Okimasu, M., Utsumi, K. (1990). "Inhibition of oxidative injury of biological membranes by astaxanthin." Physiol. Chem. Phys. Med. NMR 22(1):27-38.

Kurihara, H., Koda, H., Asami, S., Kiso, Y., Tanaka, T. (2002). "Contribution of the antioxidative property of astaxanthin to its protective effect on the promotion of cancer metastasis in mice treated with restraint stress." Life Sciences. 70(21):2509-20.

Lee, S., Bai, S., Lee, K., Namkoong, S., Na, H., Ha, K., Han, J., Yim, S., Chang, K., Kwon, Y., Lee, S., Kim, Y. (2003). "Astaxanthin Inhibits Nitric Oxide Production and Inflammatory Gene Expression by Suppressing IkB Kinase-dependent NFR-kB Activation." Molecules and Cells. 16(1):97-105.

Lee, S. et al. (1998). "Inhibition of sarcoma-180 cell-induced mouse ascites cancer by astaxanthin-containing egg yolks." J. Kor. Soc. Food Sci. Nutr. 27, 163.

Lee, S. et al. (1997). "Inhibition of benzo(a)pyrene-induced mouse forestomach neoplasia by astaxanthin containing egg yolks." Agric. Chem. Biotechnol. 40, 490.

Levy, J. et al. (2002). "Lycopene and astaxanthin inhibit human prostate cancer cell proliferation induced by androgens." Presented at 13th Int. Carotenoid Symp., Honolulu, January 6-11, 2002.

Li, W., Hellsten, A., Jacobsson, L., Blomqvist, H., Olsson, A., Yuan, X. (2004). "Alpha-tocopherol and astaxanthin decrease macrophage infiltration, apoptosis and vulnerability in atheroma of hyperlipidaemic rabbits." Journal of molecular and cellular cardiology. 37(5):969-78.

Lignell, A. (2001). "Medicament for improvement of duration of muscle function or treatment of muscle disorders or diseases." U.S. Patent #6245818.

Lignell, A., Inboor, J. (2000). "Agent for increasing the production of/in breeding and production

136

mammals." U.S. Patent #6054491.

Lignell, A., Nicolin, C., Larsson Lars-Hak. (1998). "Method for increasing the production of/in breeding and production animals in the poultry industry." U.S. Patent #5744502.

Lorenz, T. (2002). "Clinical Trial Indicates Sun Protection from BioAstin Supplement." Cyanotech Technical Bulletin based on Independent Consumer Testing Company clinical trial (unpublished). On file at Cyanotech Corporation.

Luzzano, U., Scolari, M., Grispan, M., Papi, L., Dore, J. (2003). "Haematococcus pluvialis algae meal as a natural source of astaxanthin for rainbow trout (Oncorhynchus mykiss) pigmentation." Presented at the Acquacoltura International trade show for aquaculture. Verona, Italy, October 15-17, 2003.

Lyons, N., O'Brien, N. (2002). "Modulatory effects of an algal extract containing astaxanthin on UVA-irradiated cells in culture." Journal of Dermatological Science. 30(1):73-84.

Maher, T. (2000). "Astaxanthin." Continuing Education Module, New Hope Institute of Retailing, Boulder, Colorado, "Natural Healing Track." In association with the Massachusetts College of Pharmacy and Health Sciences. August 2000.

Mahmoud, F., Haines, D., Abul, H., Abal, A., Onadeko, B., Wise, J. (2004). "In vitro effects of astaxanthin combined with ginkgolide B on T lymphocyte activation in peripheral blood mononuclear cells from asthmatic subjects." J Pharmacol Sci. 94(2):129-36.

Malila, N., Virtanen, M., Virtamo, J., Albanes, D., Pukkala, E. (2006). "Cancer incidence in a cohort of Finnish male smokers." Eur. J. Cancer Prev. 2006(15):103-107.

Malmsten, C. (1998). "Dietary Supplementation with Astaxanthin-rich Algal Meal Improves Muscle Endurance-A Double Blind Study on Male Students." Karolinska Institute, Gustavsberg, Sweden.

Martin, H., Jager, C., Ruck, C., Schimdt, M. (1999). "Anti- and Prooxidant Properties of Carotenoids." J. Prakt. Chem. 341(3):302-308.

Mason, P., Walter, M., McNulty, H., Lockwood, S., Byun, J., Day, C., Jacob, R. (2006). "Rofecoxib Increases Susceptibility of Human LDL and Membrane Lipids to Oxidative Damage: A Mechanism of Cardiotoxicity." Journal of Cardiovascular Pharmacology. 47(1):S7-S14.

Mera Pharmaceuticals, Inc. (2006). Press Release, March 14, 2006.

Mercke Odeberg, J., Lignell, A., Petterson, A., Hoglund, P. (2003). "Oral bioavailability of the antioxidant astaxanthin in humans is enhanced by incorporation of lipid based formulas." European Journal of of Pharmaceutical Sciences. 19(4):299-304.

Miyawaki, H. (2005). "Effects of astaxanthin on human blood rheology." Journal of Clinical Therapeutics & Medicines. 21(4):421-429.

Moorhead, K., Capelli, B., Cysewski, G. (2006). "Spirulina: Nature's Superfood." ISBN #0-9637511-3-1.

Mori, H., Tanaka, T., Sugie, S., Yoshimi, N., Kawamori, T., Hirose, Y., Ohnishi, M. (1997). "Chemoprevention by naturally occurring and synthetic agents in oral, liver, and large bowel carcinogenesis." Journal of Cellular Biochemestry. 27:35-41.

Murakami, C., Takemura, M., Sugiyama, Y., Kamisuki, S., Asahara, H., Kawasaki, M., Ishidoh, T., Linn, S., Yoshida, S., Sugawara, F., Yoshida, H., Sakaguchi, K., Mizushina, Y. (2002). "Vitamin A-related compounds, all-trans retinal and retinoic acids, selectively inhibit activities of mammalian replicative DNA polymerases." Biochim. Biophys. Acta. 1574, 85.

Murillo, E. (1992). "Hypercholsterolemic effect of canthaxanthin and astaxanthin in rats." Latin American Archives of Nutrition. 42(4):409-13.

Nagaki, et al. (2006). "The supplementation effect of astaxanthin on accommodation and asthenopia." Journal of Clinical Therapeutics & Medicines. 22(1):41-54.

Nagaki, Y., Hayasaka, S., Yamada, T., Hayasaka, Y., Sanada, M., Uonomi, T. (2002). "Effects of Astaxanthin on accommodation, critical flicker fusion, and pattern visual evoked potential in visual display terminal workers." Journal of Traditional Medicines. 19(5):170–173.

Naito, Y., Uchiyama, K., Mizushima, K., Kuroda, M., Akagiri, S., Takagi, T., Handa, O., Kokura, S., Yoshida, N., Ichikawa, H., Takahashi, J., Yoshikawa, T. (2006). "Microarray profiling of gene expression patterns in glomerular cells of astaxanthin-treated diabetic mice: a nutrigenomic approach." International Journal of Molecular Medicine. 18(4):685-95.

Naito, Y., Uchiyama, K., Aoi, W., Hasegawa, G., Nakamura, N., Yoshida, N., Maoka, T., Takahashi, J., Yoshikawa, T. (2004). "Prevention of diabetic nephropathy by treatment with astaxanthin in diabetic db/db mice." BioFactors. 20(1):49-59.

Nakamura, et al. (2004). "Changes in Visual Function Following Peroral Astaxanthin." Japanese Journal of Clinical Ophthalmology. 58(6):1051-1054.

Nir, Y., Spiller, G. (2002a). "BioAstin, a natural astaxanthin from microalgae, helps relieve pain and improves performance in patients with carpel tunnel syndrome (CTS)." Journal of the American College of Nutrition. 21(5):Oct, 2002.

Nir, Y., Spiller, G. (2002b). "BioAstin helps relieve pain and improves performance in patients with rheumatoid arthritis." Journal of the American College of Nutrition. 21(5):Oct, 2002.

Nishikawa, Y., Minenaka, Y., Ichimura, M., Tatsumi, K., Nadamoto, T., Urabe, K. (2005). "Effects of astaxanthin and vitamin C on the prevention of gastric ulcerations in stressed rats." Journal of nutritional science and vitaminology. 51(3):135-41.

Nishino, et al, (1999). "Cancer prevention by carotenoids." Pure & Appl. Chem. 71, 2273.

Nitta, T., Ogami, K., Shiratori, K. (2005). "The effects of Astaxanthin on Accommodation and Asthenopia—Dose Finding Study in Healthy Volunteers." Clinical Medicine. 21(5):543-556.

O'Connor I., O'Brien, N. (1998). "Modulation of UVA light-induced oxidative stress by beta carotene, lutein and astaxanthin in cultured fibroblasts." Journal of . Dermatological Science. 16(3):226-230.

Ohgami, K., Shiratori, K., Kotake, S., Nishida, T., Mizuki, N., Yazawa, K., Ohno, S. (2003). "Effects of astaxanthin on lipopolysaccharide-induced inflammation in vitro and in vivo." Investigative Ophthalmology and Visual Science. 44(6):2694-701.

Okai, Y., Higashi-Okai, K. (1996). "Possible immunomodulating activities of carotenoids in in-vitro cell culture experiments." International Journal of Immunopharmacology. 18(12):753–8.

Onogi, N., Okuno, M., Matsushima-Nishiwaki, R., Fukutomi, Y., Moriwaki, H., Muto, Y., Kojima, S. (1998). "Antiproliferative effect of carotenoids on human colon cancer cells without conversion to retinoic acid." Nutr. Cancer. 32, 20.

Oryza Oil & Fat Chemical Company. (2006). "Natural Antioxidant for Neuro-protection, Vision Enhancement & Skin Rejuvenation." September 7, 2006.

Osterlie, M., Bjerkeng, B., Liaaen-Jensen, S. (2000). "Plasma appearance and distribution of astax-anthin E/Z and R/S isomers in plasma lipoproteins of men after single dose administration of astaxanthin." Journal of Nutrition and Biochemistry. 11(10):482-90.

Perricone, N. (2006). "The Perricone Weight-Loss Diet." Pg 98-99. ISBN #0-345-48593-9.

Perry, S. (2006). "Keeping Inflammation at Bay." Today's Health and Wellness Magazine. August, 2006. Pg 54-56.

Potter, J. (1997). "Cancer prevention: epidemiology and experiment." Cancer Lett. 114, 7.

Rauscher, R., Edenharder, R., Platt, K. (1998) "In vitro antimutagenic and in vivo anticlastogenic effects of carotenoids and solvent extracts from fruits and vegetables rich in carotenoids." Mutat. Res. 413, 129.

Rock, C. (2003). "Carotenoid update." J. Am. Diet. Assoc. 103, 423.

Rousseau, E., Davison, A., Dunn, B. (1992). "Protection by beta carotene and related compounds against oxygen-mediated cytotoxicity and genotoxicity: implications for carcinogenesis and anticarcinogenesis." Free Radical Biology & Medicine. 13(4):407-33.

Savoure, N., Briand, G., Amory-Touz, M., Combre, A., Maudet, M. (1995). "Vitamin A status and metabolism of cutaneous polyamines in the hairless mouse after UV irradiation: action of

138

beta-carotene and astaxanthin." International Journal for Vitamin and Nutrition Research. 65(2):79-86.

Sawaki, K., Yoshigi, H., Aoki, K., Koikawa, N., Azumane, A., Kaneko, K., Yamaguchi, M. (2002). "Sports Performance Benefits from Taking Natural Astaxanthin Characterized by Visual Acuity and Muscle Fatigue Improvements in Humans." Journal of Clinical Therapeutics & Medicines. 18:(9)73-88.

Sears, B. (2005). "Silent Inflammation." Nutraceuticals World Magazine. May, 2005. Pg 38-45.

Setnikar, I., Senin, P., Rovati, L. (2005). "Antiatherosclerotic efficacy of policosanol, red yeast rice extract and astaxanthin in the rabbit." Arzneimittelforschung. 55(6):312-7.

Shimidzu, N., Goto, M., Miki, W. (1996). "Carotenoids as singlet oxygen quechers in marine organisms." Fisheries Science. 62(1):134-137.

Shiratori, K., Ogami, K., Nitta, T. (2005). "The effects of Astaxanthin on Accommodation and Asthenopia—Efficacy Identification Study in Healthy Volunteers." Clinical Medicine. 21(6):637-650.

Singh, G. (1998). "Recent considerations in nonsteroidal anti-inflammatory drug gastropathy." Am J Med. 105(1B):315-85.

Spiller, G., Dewell, A., Chaves, S., Rakidzich, Z. (2006a). "Effect of daily use of natural astaxanthin on C-reactive protein." On file at Cyanotech Corporation.

Spiller, G., Dewell, A., Chaves, S., Rakadzich, Z. (2006b). "Effect of daily use of natural astaxanthin on symptoms associated with Tennis Elbow (lateral humeral epicondylitis). On file at Cyanotech Corporation.

Sun, S. et al. (1998). "Anti-tumor activity of astaxanthin on Meth-A tumor cells and its mode of action." FASEB J. 12, A966.

Suzuki, Y., Ohgami, K., Shiratori, K., Jin, X., Ilieva, I., Koyama, Y., Yazawa. K., Yoshida, K., Kase, S., Ohno, S. (2006). "Suppressive effects of astaxanthin against rat endotoxin-induced uveitis by inhibiting the NF-kappaB signaling pathway." Experimental Eye Research. 82(2):275-81.

Takahashi, J., Kajita. (2005). "Effects of astaxanthin on accommodative recovery." Journal of Clinical Therapeutics & Medicines. 21(4):431-436.

Tanaka, T., Kawamori, T., Ohnishi, M., Makita, H., Mori, H., Satoh, K., Hara, A. (1995a). "Suppression of azomethane-induced rat colon carcinogenesis by dietary administration of naturally occurring xanthophylls astaxanthin and canthaxanthin during the postinitiation phase." Carcinogenesis. 16(12):2957-63.

Tanaka, T., Makita, H., Ohnishi, M., Mori, H., Satoh, K., Hara, A. (1995b). "Chemoprevention of rat oral carcinogenesis by naturally occurring xanthophylls, astaxanthin and canthaxanthin." Cancer Research. 55(18):4059-64.

Tanaka, T., Morishita, Y., Suzui, M., Kojima, T., Okumura, A., Mori, H. (1994). "Chemoprevention of mouse urinary bladder carcinogenesis by the naturally occurring carotenoids astaxanthin." Carcinogenesis. 15(1):15-19.

Thibodeau, A., Lauzier, E. (2003). "Dietary/Nutritional Supplements: The New Ally to Topical Cosmetic Formulations." Cosmetics & Toiletries Magazine, January 2003. 118(1):57-64.

Tomita, Y., Jyonouchi, H., Engelman, R., Day, N., Good, R. (1993). "Preventive action of carotenoids on the development of lymphadenopathy and proteinuria in MRL-lpr/lpr mice." Autoimmunity. 16(2):95-102.

Trimeks Company Study (2003). On file at Cyanotech Corporation.

Tso, M., Lam, T. (1996) "Method of Retarding and Ameliorating Central Nervous System and Eye Damage." U.S. Patent #5527533.

Turujman, S., Warner, W., Wei, R., Albert, R. (1997). "Rapid liquid chromatographic method to distinguish wild salmon from aquacultured salmon fed synthetic astaxanthin." J. AOAC Int. 80:622-632.

Uchiyama, K., Naito, Y., Hasegawa, G., Nakamura, N., Takahashi, J., Yoshikawa, T. (2002).

139

"Astaxanthin protects b-cells against glucose toxicity in diabetic db/db mice." Redox Report. 7(5):290-3.

Underwood, A. (2005). "Quieting a Body's Defenses." Newsweek Magazine, "Special Summer Issue," August 2005. Pg. 26-28.

Waagbo, R., Hamre, K., Bjerkas, E., Berge, R., Wathne, E., Lie, O., Torstensen, B. (2003). "Cataract formation in Atlantic salmon, Salmo salar L., smolt relative to dietary pro- and antioxidants and lipid level." Journal of Fish Diseases. 26(4):213-29.

Wang, X., Willen, R., Wadstrom, T. (2000). "Astaxanthin-rich algal meal and vitamin C inhibit Helicobacter pylori infection in BALB/cA mice." Antimicrobial Agents and Chemotherapy. 44(9):2452-7.

Wargovich, M. (1997). "Experimental evidence for cancer preventive elements in food." Cancer Lett. 114, 11.

Watanabe, T., Vassallo-Auis, R. (2003). "Broodstock nutrition research on marine finfish in Japan." Aquaculture. 227(1-4):35-61.

Witt, E., Reznick, C., Viguie, P., Starke-Reed, P., Packer, L. (1992). "Exercise, oxidative damage and effects on antioxidant manipulation." J. Nutr. 122:766-773.

Wolfe, M., Lichtensteein, D., Singh, G. (1999). "Gastrointestinal toxicity on nonsteroidal anti-inflammatory drugs." N Engl J Med. 340(24):1888-89.

Wu, T., Liao, J., Hou, W., Huang, F., Maher, T., Hu, C. (2006). "Astaxanthin protects against oxidative stress and calcium-induced porcine lens protein degradation." Journal Agriculture Food Chemistry. 54, 6:2418-23.

Wu, T, et al. (2002). "An astaxanthin-containing algal extract attenuates selenite-induced nuclear cataract formation in rat pups." Experimental Biology, 2002.

Yamashita, E. (2002). "Cosmetic Benefit of Dietary Supplements Containing Astaxanthin and Tocotrienol on Human Skin." Food Style. 21 6(6):112-17.

Yang, Z. et al. (1997). "Protective effect of astaxanthin on the promotion of cancer metastases in mice treated with restraint-stress." J. Jpn. Soc. Nutr. Food Sci. 50, 423.

Yasunori, N, et al. (2005). "The effect of astaxanthin on retinal capillary blood flow in normal volunteers." J. Clin. Ther. Med. 21(5):537-542.

Zhang, S. et al. (1999). "Dietary carotenoids and vitamins A, C, and E and risk of breast cancer." J. Natl. Cancer Inst. 91, 547

Order Form

Additional copies of this book may be ordered directly from the Publisher, Cyanotech Corporation. Please contact us by e-mail at info@cyanotech.com or by telephone at 800.395.1353 or 808.326.1353. Also, you can mail this form along with payment (please make checks payable to Cyanotech) to:

Cyanotech Corporation
73-4460 Queen Kaahumanu Hwy, Suite 102
Kailua-Kona, HI 96740 USA

Pricing is based on the volume of books purchased:

1 copy	$6.95
2 – 5 copies	$6.25
6 – 10 copies	$5.22
11 – 20 copies	$4.51
21 – 30 copies	$4.17
31 – 40 copies	$3.82
41 – 50 copies	$3.48
More than 50 copies	Please contact us for pricing

No charge for shipping.

Name: _____

Address:_____

City: _____ State: _____ Zip Code: _____

Country:_____ Telephone #: (_____)_____

Number of copies: _____ Price per copy: _____ Total: _____

ABOUT THE AUTHORS

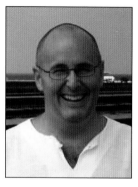

Bob Capelli has dedicated most of his professional career to natural healing and herbology. After graduating from Rutgers University with a degree in liberal arts, Bob spent four years traveling and working in developing countries in Asia and Latin America while he was in his twenties. It was during his travels that Bob developed an interest in and a deep respect for the medicinal power of plants. Upon returning to the United States, Bob began working in the natural supplement and herb industry, where he has remained for the last sixteen years.

Bob realized his dream job five years ago when he joined Cyanotech Corporation, allowing him to work with the world's premier producer of products from microalgae. Bob considers himself a living testimonial to the health benefits of Natural Astaxanthin and Spirulina—since beginning to take them on a daily basis five years ago, he has never had a cold or flu or missed a day of work!

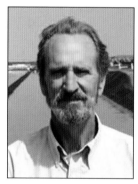

Dr. Gerald Cysewski is recognized as a world authority on microalgae. He has over thirty years experience in microalgae research and commercial production of microalgae products. His work on microalgae in 1976 was supported by the National Science Foundation at the University of California at Santa Barbara where he was an assistant professor in the department of Chemical & Nuclear Engineering He carried on his work at Battelle Northwest as group leader of microalgae research.

Dr. Cysewski co-founded Cyanotech Corporation in 1983 in Washington State. He initially served as the Company's Scientific Director and became President and CEO of Cyanotech in 1990. As the Company's Scientific Director he sought the optimum site to launch commercial production of microalgae and found the Kona coast of Hawaii, a region with abundant sunlight virtually year-round, a ready source of pure water from island aquifers, deep-ocean seawater nearby to fuel a new chill-drying technology, and access to transportation and skilled labor. Cyanotech's location combined with its advanced technology has made it the premier producer of microalgae in the world.

Dr. Cysewski holds a Bachelor of Science in Chemical Engineering from the University of Washington and a Doctorate in Chemical Engineering from the University of California at Berkeley.